AUTISTIC MENOPAUSE

A Guide to the Menopausal Transition for Autistic People and Those Supporting Them

RACHEL MOSELEY and JULIE GAMBLE-TURNER

Illustrated by Rose Matthews

Jessica Kingsley Publishers
London and Philadelphia

First published in Great Britain in 2026 by Jessica Kingsley Publishers
An imprint of John Murray Press

1

The information contained in this book is not intended to
replace the services of trained medical professionals or to be a
substitute for medical advice. You are advised to consult a doctor
on any matters relating to your health, and in particular on any
matters that may require diagnosis or medical attention.

Content Warning: This book mentions mental health and suicide.

A CIP catalogue record for this title is available from
the British Library and the Library of Congress

ISBN 978 1 80501 0 975
eISBN 978 1 80501 0 982

Printed and bound in Great Britain by Clays Ltd

Jessica Kingsley Publishers' policy is to use papers that are natural,
renewable and recyclable products and made from wood grown in
sustainable forests. The logging and manufacturing processes are expected
to conform to the environmental regulations of the country of origin.

Jessica Kingsley Publishers
Carmelite House
50 Victoria Embankment
London EC4Y 0DZ

www.jkp.com

John Murray Press
Part of Hodder & Stoughton Ltd
An Hachette Company

The authorised representative in the EEA is Hachette Ireland,
8 Castlecourt Centre, Dublin 15, D15 XTP3, Ireland (email: info@hbgi.ie)

To our research participants who asked for autistic stories of menopause, and the autistic experts who so generously and courageously shared their experiences. This is for you, for those following in your footsteps, and for those who walked this way in the darkness without the light that comes with understanding.

Acknowledgements

We humbly thank our families, friends and colleagues for their encouragement and support throughout the writing of this book. We are also so grateful to the many individuals and organizations who have supported our work on this topic and to Beyond Reflections for reviewing Chapter 11. We are particularly grateful to Henpicked: Menopause in the Workplace for actively appreciating our early research and funding our ongoing work. Last but by no means least, our sincere gratitude goes to all the autistic experts who have so generously and courageously shared their experiences of menopause for this book, and to those who participated in our research: you have taught us so much.

Contents

Introduction 9

**Part 1: Understanding menopause and the
backdrop to autistic experiences**

1. Autistic experts: 'What we wish we had known before
   going through menopause' 19

2. The biology of menopause: What's happening and what
   are those hormones playing at? 24

3. 'The change' and how it affects body and mind 33

4. The psychology of menopause: What factors can
   influence the way you experience menopause? 41

5. Why does menopause matter?: Relationships between
   menopause and health. 51

Part 2: Autistic and menopausal: The 'double whammy'

6. Autistic experts: 'If I could use one word to describe my
   experience of menopause' 62

7. Why might menopause be harder for autistic people?. . . . 66

8. The bigger picture: Autistic people navigating midlife. . . . 80

9. The importance of knowing: When menopause comes
   before an autism diagnosis 89

10. Menopause and other forms of neurodivergence:
Learning disabilities, ADHD and AuDHD 98

11. Multiply marginalized: Experiences from ethnic, sex and
gender minorities 108

Part 3: Autistic experiences of menopause

12. Physical changes: The expected and the unexpected. 118

13. Emotional changes: Mood, coping, stress and distress . . . 128

14. Attention, memory and other thought processes:
Changes and their impact on everyday living and work . . . 139

15. Communication changes and their impact on
relationships 150

16. Sensory changes and their impact at menopause. 161

Part 4: Managing menopause

17. Autistic experts: 'Advice for autistic people about
navigating menopause?' 172

18. Positives of menopause...?! 185

19. Life on the other side of menopause: Postmenopausal
experiences 194

20. What should professionals supporting autistic people
through menopause be aware of? 201

21. Conclusion: Looking to the future (where are we now
and where do we need to go?) 213

Resources 216

Key points for professionals 218

Endnotes 220

Index 247

Introduction

Dear reader,

The warmest of welcomes to you. It is somewhat daunting writing this preface; at the same time, it feels like a great honour, knowing that just a little way in the future, we will be connecting with you through this book. We are so happy that you have joined us here and will journey with us through these pages.

Who are we, and why did we write this book?

We are academics in psychology, and we conduct research on a range of different topics. Dr Rachel Moseley started out 13 years ago looking at differences between autistic and non-autistic brains, but now specializes in the mental health of autistic adults. Professor Julie Gamble-Turner has over 30 years of experience studying the impact of stressful life experiences and hormone changes on physical health and wellbeing across the lifespan. Back in 2018, we joined forces to conduct the first research study investigating autistic experiences of menopause, bringing together our different academic backgrounds and professional training. Between us, we also brought a multitude of relevant lived experiences, including the challenges of receiving an adult autism diagnosis and the turbulence of menopause.

Our initial project on autistic menopause was done on a shoe-string budget, undertaken as part of an MSc course by a (splendid) student, Ms Tanya Druce. We had no idea that we would find a total absence of information about autistic menopause, and moreover, what appeared to be an immense need in autistic people who were suffering from this lack of information and awareness. Our ongoing research, and this book, are all aimed at trying to address that need.

Who are you, and what do we hope you will take from this book?

Perhaps you work with autistic people. Thank you for your dedication to those you work with, which has led you to try to find out more about autistic experiences of menopause. Our intention is that this book will help you to help others. Towards that goal, this book brings together key context, relevant research, and the most important source of learning: lived experiences of autistic experts. The whole book is written to be useful to you, and there is direct advice for supporting autistic people in professional contexts, such as health and social care, in Chapter 20. If you're short on time and need the 'TL;DR' (too long; didn't read) version, you can find this in 'Key points for professionals' at the end of the book (page 216).

Perhaps you are the loved one of someone who is autistic. Thank you, likewise, for trying to learn more so that you can support that person. We have written this book to help you know what to expect before menopause happens, to help you empathize, understand and support your loved one.

Perhaps you are autistic and preparing to enter menopause; autistic and going through menopause; or autistic and postmenopausal. Perhaps you are wondering if you're autistic but don't know for sure; perhaps you are searching for an explanation for why life has always been hard, and why menopause is proving such a struggle. To you we extend our deepest welcome, and our intention is that you will find clarity, self-understanding, comfort and connection with others who have had similar experiences. This book should empower you to have important conversations with those around you, including your loved ones and professionals who might be in a position to help you (and to that end, you should find Chapter 20 and perhaps also the 'Key points for professionals' at the end of the book helpful, too!).

The experience of being autistic is sadly often that of feeling disconnected from other people, lost in a world you don't understand and where you don't fit in. It's like trying to act in a play where everybody but you knows the script. Unfortunately, going through menopause can also be like this for some autistic people. Strikingly, one phrase has emerged again and again across the many autistic people who have talked to us about menopause:

" 'I thought I was going mad!'

They often follow this up with statements like:

" 'What I'm experiencing is nothing like what people describe when they talk about menopause.'

" 'What's going on?'

" 'What's wrong with me?'

In this book, we hope to tell you (spoiler alert):

- You are not going mad.
- If your menopause seems harder than that of other people, that is not your fault. There are numerous reasons why your menopause might be more difficult than that of others.
- There are treatments, and there is a way through. If you are in the midst of menopausal symptoms right now, how you're feeling at this moment is not how you will feel forever.

You don't need to take our word for it. In this book, we have brought together 16 experts on autistic menopause – autistic people who have experienced or are currently experiencing menopausal symptoms (henceforth referred to as our 'autistic experts', since they are experts by experience). Their stories are embedded throughout the book. You will hear about the kinds of changes and symptoms they experienced during menopause, and how these impacted their lives. Most importantly, you will hear their thoughts from the other side of menopause, and their advice about getting through it and seeking help. If you are not yet menopausal, this book will give you some idea about what you might experience when that time comes. And it will help you to have some important conversations with the people around you, so that they are ready to support you.

Again and again, we've witnessed the relief expressed by our research participants when they could finally talk about their menopause and hear the experiences of other autistic people. Having felt so alone, they were able to hear the feelings of confusion, lostness and difference shared by others, swap strategies that worked for them, and feel connected to a wider community. In difficult times, a book can be a doorway to connection and belonging. We cannot bring you together physically, but we hope this book reassures you that you are not mad, and you are not alone.

What you will find in this book

This book is divided into four parts; here is an overview of what each will cover.

Part 1

In the first part, we will be laying the foundations for the rest of this book: in order to understand why menopause might be challenging for autistic people, we need to understand it in its full complexity. In this first part, we'll explore two sides of a two-way relationship: how menopause impacts brain, mind and body, as well as how the person's psychological state, life experiences and health affect how they experience menopause. We'll also consider why menopause matters, and indeed why it needs to be taken seriously and supported.

Part 2

In the second part of the book, we'll build on those earlier foundations by showing their relevance in an autistic context. Where Part 1 shows how extensively menopause affects brain, mind and body, Part 2 considers how autistic people might already differ in these aspects. Where Part 1 shows how strongly menopause is influenced by our health and life experiences, such that it varies greatly from individual to individual, Part 2 will consider how characteristics and life experiences common to autistic people might give rise to difficulties during menopause. We'll explore issues and challenges that might more likely be faced by autistic people, such as entering menopause without crucial bits of information about your neurodivergent self or having other marginalized identities.

Part 3

In the third part of the book, we'll speak at greater length about the different symptoms and changes that autistic people experience during menopause. We'll start with how autistic people experience the physical changes of menopause. We'll then think about four important areas where autistic people differ from non-autistic people – their emotions, cognitive processes, communication and relationships, and sensory experiences – and consider how these are impacted by menopause.

Part 4

As we draw to a close in the fourth part of our book, we'll talk about how autistic people cope with menopause, with a lot of helpful advice from our experts. Because hoping for brighter times on the horizon is an important aspect of coping, we will hear from our experts about the positive growth and silver linings they experienced on account of going through menopause, and about their lives post-menopause. Finally, we'll explore ways that professionals can help autistic people cope during menopause, and conclude with actions for those in positions with the power to change things.

A few things to bear in mind as you read this book

Menopause is different for everyone. Throughout this book, you will quickly see how variable menopause is, for autistic and non-autistic people alike. Undoubtedly, some autistic people go through menopause with no difficulties at all. One thing we have learnt as researchers is that people who struggle with something are understandably much more likely to want to talk about it. This means that we have mostly talked to people who have been struggling with menopause, since autistic people with only very minor menopause symptoms were unlikely to think it was worth talking about! This is so important because we do not want you to come away from this book frightened, thinking that your experience of menopause will definitely look like some of the more difficult ones described in this book. You might have no difficulties at all, given the huge variation that exists.

People use different language to talk about menopause. We'll typically use the word 'menopause' in a collective way to encapsulate the time when people are experiencing menopausal symptoms: this includes the phase called perimenopause, as well as the 'passing' or 'reaching' of menopause and into postmenopause when people are still symptomatic (see Chapter 2 for more on these terms and stages). We've tried to be as consistent as possible, so where we write 'menopause', you know we're talking about the whole symptomatic process from perimenopause into early postmenopause when people are still experiencing symptoms. We talk about 'menopausal autistic people', similarly, to describe autistic people who are experiencing menopausal symptoms, though they might be at different stages of the process. When we are talking about symptoms or experiences characteristic of certain stages of menopause, we'll refer to that stage specifically, for example, perimenopause (where we might refer to people being 'perimenopausal'), or postmenopause (where we'll talk about people being 'postmenopausal', and if it's relevant, highlight whether we mean the earlier symptomatic stages or the later postmenopause years when symptoms abate). Our autistic experts, likewise, usually use the terms 'menopause' and sometimes 'the menopause' to refer to the symptomatic time from perimenopause through into postmenopause, except in places where they're talking about specific stages of the menopausal transition. We have kept as much of their original wording as possible.

Different kinds of minds enrich the world we live in. Autism is just one of those forms of natural neurological diversity: a difference in the way the brain works, which gives rise to a totally different experience of the world. For many, being autistic is also an important part of their personal and social identity, something that makes them part of a larger community of autistic people.[1] Autistic people differ in the ways they think, feel and talk about their autism, and we utterly respect their right to do so. That said, research suggests that seeing autism through the lens of words like 'deficit' or 'disorder' only reinforces unhealthy, unhappy self-perceptions in autistic people, suggesting they are broken or deficient.[2] As such, we encourage professionals to align themselves with a neurodiversity framework as their default position.[3] For this reason, and because it is the preference of autistic people who respond to surveys, we will use identity-first language throughout this book ('autistic person', rather than 'person with autism'). We will also talk about menopause experiences of autistic people, rather than autistic women, since not all autistic people who experience menopause are women moreover, since some intersex people also experience menopause, not all those who experience menopause were assigned female at birth. This book focuses on menopause in people who were assigned female at birth, and the experience of menopause is quite different for people who do not identify as women. Those going through menopause who are not women have very specific difficulties and needs. While they are not the focus of this book, the intersection of autism, gender divergence and menopause is an important one for professionals to be aware of (and we'll come back to it in Chapter 11, page 112).

Part 1

UNDERSTANDING MENOPAUSE AND THE BACKDROP TO AUTISTIC EXPERIENCES

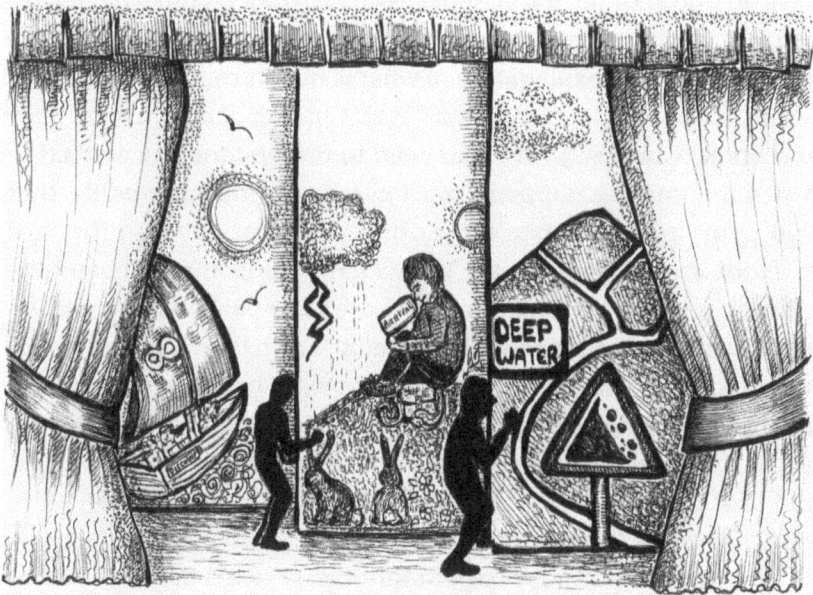

In the first part of this book, we want to set the scene for both menopause and autism, before bringing together these two areas throughout the rest of the book. At first, these two topics might seem to be a rather niche combination, or to the uninitiated perhaps a puzzling intersection. Yet if you or someone you know or care for are autistic and have been through or are going through menopause, then you are probably aware that the topic is far from niche.

The topic of menopause, and the topic of autism in people assigned female at birth, have something in common. Until recently, both have individually received relatively little attention; when combined, even less. In fact, together they had been given no academic attention at all, until we published the first work on this a few years ago.[1] Thankfully the experience of menopause for autistic people, and neurodivergent people more generally, is now emerging as a topic of particular interest. The reason for this is that autistic features and the experiences of autistic people tap into key features of menopause and menopausal symptoms. In fact, we would go as far as to suggest that menopause and autism can have a reciprocal relationship, and that for autistic people going through menopause, it is possible that a spiral of effects or experiences emerges.

To understand the combined effect that menopause and autism have on one another, it is first necessary to understand what menopause is. We'll start by demystifying the menopausal transition with a description and explanation of what is meant by menopause, and whats happening at a hormonal level (Chapter 2) and in your body and brain (Chapter 3). We also need to understand the context in which menopause happens, most commonly during midlife, that mid-point in the lifespan most often viewed as between the ages of about 40 and 65 years; the events happening at midlife and the influences on them at that time can have an impact on the way a person experiences menopause (Chapter 4). From there we look at why menopause matters and the links that exist between menopause and health, taking a lifespan approach. In doing this we consider the impact of stress experienced before midlife and during menopause, and how these impact on health both during menopause and also going forwards in the lifespan as we age (Chapter 5). Throughout, as we outline the landscape of menopause, we'll flag up specific clues that lead us to understand why menopause might present particular difficulties for autistic (or otherwise neurodivergent) people. We start in the first chapter with some compelling words from our autistic experts: what they wished they had known before going through menopause.

Chapter 1

Autistic experts

'What we wish we had known before
going through menopause'

66 'I wish I'd known everything about the menopause, and not just that it was
a hot flush.' CLAIRE

66 'I wish I'd known about the physical changes... weight and ballooning,
water retention and changes in your body... the cognitive difficulties.' ANN

66 'I wish I'd known that it wasn't just stuff like hot flushes... the emotional
effects were far worse, far more debilitating, and the effect on sleep."'
KATIE

66 'I wish I'd known the other things, like the sheer amount of anxiety and
effect on my senses.' LILY

66 'I wish I'd known about loss of libido; mood swings; that HRT can cause
problems.' SALLY

66 'I wish I'd known I was autistic/neurodivergent.' BRIDIE, LILY, SUZI AND
JANET

66 'I wish I'd known it started so early and... that HRT is a good thing.' ALICE

66 'I wish I'd known more about alternatives to HRT... before I started taking
it.' SPIKE

66 'I wish I'd known how little other people know, especially doctors.' DAISY

" 'I wish I'd known what I could do... to mitigate the symptoms...' TARA

" 'I wish I had kept my Mirena [coil] in, as the HRT wasn't a huge success. Also teeth loss, I never knew about that being a side effect.' FLORENCE

" 'I would have liked to have known that it's actually not that uncommon for women to go into menopause in their early 40s.' ANNE

" 'A lot more about menopause and exactly what it entails.' BASSAI SHO

" '[that I was] in for a bit of a ride.' THE CAT

In this sample of quotes from our autistic experts, it is clear that they felt there was a lot they did not know about menopause before they experienced it. There is a definite sense of feeling unprepared and lacking the necessary information in advance of entering menopause, as has been found in research on menopause more generally[1] and as we and others have found consistently across a number of studies with autistic people.[2] Lacking the necessary information meant that people struggled to make sense of the symptoms they were experiencing at menopause, and they were unable to seek the help they needed. Autistic participants in research studies have emphasized the need for scientific information about menopause delivered in an accessible way,[3] which is what we hope this book will give you.

Onset and duration of menopause

Many of our experts described wishing that they had been more aware of when menopause might start, to avoid being taken unawares by it starting earlier or more suddenly than they had anticipated. Anne mentioned that she would have found it helpful to have 'known that it's actually not that uncommon for women to go into menopause in their early 40s'. It is actually perfectly normal for people to enter the first stages of menopause (called perimenopause) at this age, but this was not communicated even by Anne's doctor when she sought help for symptoms. How many years menopause symptoms would last was also something many of our experts were unaware of before entering menopause. Some had expected it to last a couple of years and wished they had known that 'the symptoms could go on for 20-plus years' (Bridie).

Range and severity of menopausal symptoms

Many talked about wishing they had known the full range of symptoms associated with menopause, beyond hot flushes/flashes or stereotypical forgetfulness and being 'just a bit ditzy' (Ann). They talked about being unaware of the extent of symptoms, of the full range of effects on the body and the brain, including biological, psychological and cognitive symptoms. Some mentioned unexpected menopausal symptoms such as pain in their joints, personality changes, dental problems, and underlying conditions such as diabetes and heart disease emerging at menopause. They also talked about the unanticipated severity of symptoms, wishing they had known 'how bad hot flushes could be' and 'the sheer amount of anxiety' (Lily) – particularly with the compounding impact of ongoing health conditions making the experience 'overwhelming' (Daisy).

More preparation, information, education and awareness

The call for more preparation, education, information and awareness about menopause abounded in the comments from our autistic experts. A desire to have more information about menopause much earlier in life was also voiced; it was suggested that just as information about puberty is taught, so too menopause should be talked about and discussed from an early age as part of education about life, to 'not go in as blind as I did' (Bassai Sho). In particular, our experts frequently mentioned wishing they had known more about hormone replacement therapy (HRT), some wishing they had known more about its health benefits and others wishing to have had more information about its possible side effects or that it may not suit everyone. Lack of information meant that people were often left feeling frightened or as if they were going 'completely mad' (Lily). This was made worse by not knowing where to go or where to reach out for help and understanding and being faced with a lack of support when they did seek medical help. Some mentioned wishing they had known in advance about alternative treatments for menopause symptoms, such as acupuncture, that they had since found helpful. We'll share more of the things that helped our experts cope during menopause in Chapter 17.

Knowing neurodivergent status and diagnosis

Most of our autistic experts specified that they wished they had known about their neurodivergent status at the time of going through menopause, with some saying they wished they'd known this 'above all else' (Lily). Not knowing at the time had made it difficult to understand the intensity of emotions such as anxiety that they had experienced, and the impact of menopause on their sensory sensitivities. They felt that having known about what was normal for an autistic person would have meant they could seek support and understanding; been reassured their experiences were normal. As one of our experts described it:

> 'I really wish I'd known, and that there was somebody who could have sat down and explained to me, that "all these things that you've got, is autism. And then when you start to go through the menopause, it might just be like this a little bit".' SUZI

Others mentioned wishing they could have disentangled what was menopause and what was autism, to help them identify what was going on and how to cope with the different experiences. Some of our experts talked about the intensity of the combined effect of autism and menopause without being able to make sense of what was happening, and the impact this had on them personally, socially and professionally (for instance, in friend and family relationships, and with some losing their jobs).

This is what our autistic experts beautifully articulated that they wished they had known before they went into menopause. Their advice touches on many of the key elements of menopause and health in midlife, and it also starts to suggest some issues of particular concern for autistic people.

In the next few chapters, we rewind a little to consider the details of what menopause is, the physical, psychological and midlife changes of menopause, and why the experience of menopause matters. It is crucial to do this to fully understand how and why menopause might present a particular challenge to autistic people, and even more importantly, understand what can be done to support autistic people during menopause, to ultimately improve their health and wellbeing.

Chapter 2

The biology of menopause

What's happening and what are those hormones playing at?

Menopause is

Puberty in reverse

What is menopause?

Menopause is, in biological terms, a change in reproductive hormone levels, taking a person from a reproductive state to a non-reproductive one. From a medical or scientific point of view, menopause is defined as 'the permanent cessation of menstrual cycles following the loss of ovarian follicular activity',[1] and a person is referred to as having reached menopause at the point when their periods have ceased for at least 12 months. Menopause has frequently been described as 'puberty in reverse', which in many ways is quite appropriate. Puberty is more openly discussed and less stigmatized than menopause but has the similarity of being another hormonal transition point in the lifespan, one which marks the transition into adolescence. Just like puberty, which for people with ovaries can be seen as starting with their first period, menopause is both a process, as it happens over time (across a number of years), and also marked by a specific moment in time (very precisely it is the day that marks exactly 12 months after a person's periods have stopped; at this point we say a person has 'passed' or 'reached' menopause, and from thereon they're technically 'postmenopausal', although menopausal symptoms continue for some time as you'll see in Chapter 19). In fact, the process of menopause really does mirror puberty in many ways, in respect of what is happening biologically as well as some similarity in its physical and emotional effects.

Why do we go through menopause?

In thinking about what menopause is, it's worth considering just briefly the interesting fact that apart from humans, menopause occurs in very few non-human animals. This makes it quite a unique and special phenomenon. So far it has only been observed in five species of female whale, including the killer whale,[2] and in female Ngogo chimpanzees in the wild.[3] This begs the question: why does it happen?[4] Why don't animals just keep their reproductive ability for the whole of their lives, so that they can pass on more of their genes?

From an evolutionary perspective, various hypotheses exist by way of explanation. Evidence suggests that these particular mammals (us included) can live relatively long lives, so they have time for post-reproductive survival (life continuing beyond being fertile). More than this, though, the reason seems to lie in a combination of family-related factors. First, the older female is able to provide help and support to younger family members, particularly those who are raising their offspring (known as the mother and grandmother hypotheses).[5] Second, it also avoids conflict for resources which would happen if the older females were to continue reproducing at the same time as their daughters (the conflict hypothesis), particularly as the offspring of the younger generations usually do better in these scenarios.[6]

These evolutionary explanations for menopause help us understand the significance it has for survival; to maximize intergenerational benefit and minimize intergenerational harm.[7] Of course, we humans have a complex psychological, social and cultural existence that sets us apart from other animals, but the occurrence of menopause in non-human animals suggests that it has an important evolutionary reason and purpose, perhaps shining a more positive light on self-worth, importance and fulfilment postmenopause.

Understanding and defining menopause

So, let's go back to humans, armed with the insight that menopause is relatively unique and of special importance. What else do we know about it? Most people have at least a vague understanding of what menopause is: a point in the lifespan at which a woman's hormones decline, and they go through a period of having hot flushes and mood swings. But compared to general understanding of that other reproductive transition point, puberty, menopause knowledge is relatively low,[8] particularly in young adults who are premenopausal.[9] Even in scientific writing, there is a lot of inconsistency in the way different stages of menopause are defined.[10]

Thankfully, we do have an accepted definition of the different reproductive stages throughout the lifespan, known as STRAW+10 (the Stages of Reproductive Aging Workshop + 10). Originally developed back in 2001, it was revised ten years on to be more inclusive and relevant to all people assigned female at birth, whatever their age, ethnicity, social and financial status, weight or body mass index (BMI), lifestyle factors (e.g. amount of exercise or smoking), and current and historic health conditions (e.g. cancer, or irregular menstrual cycles).[11] Importantly, the STRAW+10 criteria allow us to differentiate between the effects of ovarian ageing (i.e. menopause) and those associated with ageing more generally.[12] This is important since it shines a light on which particular illnesses can be treated and how. For instance, if we know that certain health issues are related to menopause, it gives us a good clue that the hormonal changes might be at the root of the problem and so treatment might involve increasing levels of those dwindling hormones. We'll come back to this later, as it's an important distinction when it comes to preventing illness and protecting your health in the future. So, with these stages in mind, let's take a closer look at the reproductive transitions experienced by people assigned female at birth.

Menopause situated within the reproductive lifespan

STRAW+10 describes seven key stages of reproductive ageing in women and people assigned female at birth. The first three make up the early, peak and late **reproductive stages**, starting with the first period and continuing through until periods become increasingly and persistently irregular.[13] In other descriptions of menopause, this time is also sometimes known as **premenopause**, when a person is in a reproductive state and their menstrual cycle is still regular. At the point where periods become increasingly irregular, we enter the **menopausal transition**, which spans a couple of stages (early to late menopausal transition) and continues until the final menstrual period (although, of course, a person won't know it's their final period until, over time, they have no further periods). **Perimenopause**, according to STRAW+10, straddles the menopausal transition (when periods are persistently irregular) and runs into the start of **postmenopause** (marked by 12 months in a row without a period). Incidentally, although not considered to be in the reproductive phase, people can remain fertile during perimenopause, although fertility is significantly declining at this time. It's worth bearing in mind that the onset of perimenopause can be difficult to diagnose since blood tests can be misleading due to the fluctuation in hormones; it is usually on the basis of symptoms that perimenopause is indicated. Postmenopause describes the two final menopausal stages (early to late postmenopause), to the point at which reproductive hormones remain low and are relatively stable throughout the rest of the lifespan.

When it comes to the language that non-scientists use about menopause, you'll hear a lot of different things. Some people, like us, use the simple phrase 'menopause' (or the menopausal transition) to cover the whole of that symptomatic time including perimenopause, the point of passing or reaching menopause, and those early postmenopause years when symptoms are still bothersome; when we're talking specifically about postmenopause, we try to highlight whether people are postmenopausal and still symptomatic, or post-menopausal in later years when symptoms have abated. However, you will sometimes hear people talk about stages like 'perimeno-pause' specifically (as do we, in parts of this book). As these symp-tomatic stages blend into one another, we feel it is more inclusive to use a phrase which covers the whole time when people are expe-riencing menopausal symptoms. At an individual level, though, it is often very important for people to know whether they are perimeno-pausal, have reached menopause, or are postmenopausal.

The hormone changes happening throughout these various reproductive, menopausal transition, perimenopause and post-menopause stages are associated with different types and severity of symptoms. It's common for menopausal symptoms to continue into postmenopause, as we'll talk more about later. Figure 2.1 illus-trates some of these reproductive terms.

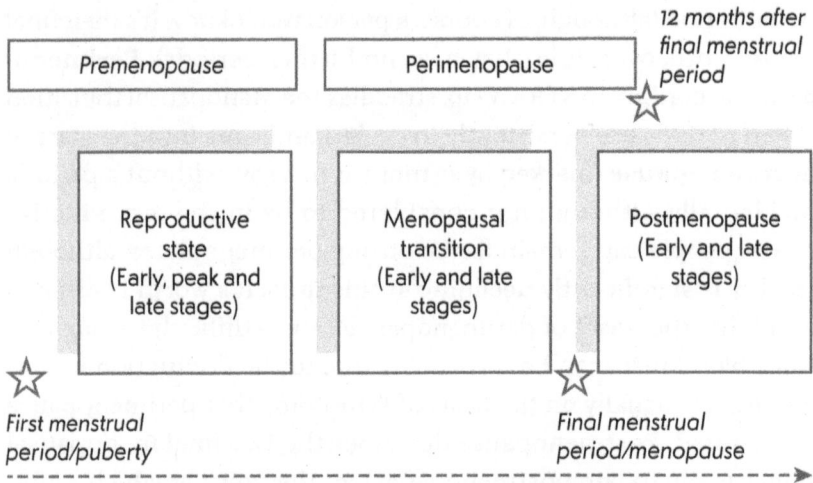

Figure 2.1 Common terms across the reproductive lifespan and key menopausal stages

Menopause is often known as 'the change' or 'the change of life'. People with ovaries make up approximately 50% of the world's population, and they can all expect to experience menopause at some point in their life – but that's about where the certainty ends. There's currently no definitive way for people to know when their menopause will begin, how long it'll last, what symptoms they'll experience and how severe these will be. Unfortunately, not even doctors can tell you these things.

There are, however, some clues about the age at which an individual's menopause will naturally begin and how long it will last, based on a number of sociodemographic and personal factors: for example we know that genetics explains about 50% of the differences seen in age at menopause,[14] and ethnicity, socioeconomic status and lifestyle also influence this[15] (more about these in Chapters 3, 4 and 5). The length of time that menopause lasts and the symptoms experienced vary enormously between people. In fact, different scientific sources note varying lengths of time for each phase of menopause and the whole of the menopausal process itself, showing just how varied it is. On average, though, perimenopause begins between a person's mid to late 40s and lasts approximately four to ten years.[16] The average age at which women and people with ovaries reach menopause (that point when periods have ceased for 12 consecutive months) also varies between countries and geographical regions of the world, but is usually between ages 47 and 51 years.[17] Evidence suggests that people in African, Latin American, Asian and Middle Eastern countries reach natural menopause earliest, while those in Europe, Australia and the USA reach menopause later.[18] The more educated a person and the higher their level of occupation, the later their age of reaching menopause; in those who smoked, menopause occurs earlier.[19]

Menopause reached between the ages of 40 and 45 years is termed **early menopause** and happens in about 5% of women and people with ovaries.[20] When menopause occurs even earlier, before 40 years of age, it is considered **premature menopause** or **premature ovarian failure**[21] (also referred to as premature ovarian insufficiency or primary ovarian insufficiency – POI). This happens to about 1% of women and people with ovaries, either spontaneously or induced through surgery or medical treatment.[22] While our focus in this book is on natural menopause, which tends to happen in the earlier part of the midlife years, we acknowledge those who go into menopause earlier in life. This brings its own particular challenges, which we would certainly not want to overlook, but many of the points we make throughout this book will still be relevant to those who experience menopause at this younger age.

What's going on? A look behind the scenes at menopause

If we examine what's happening at a biological level during the process of menopause, there are two main interacting systems that undergo complex changes. These involve hormones produced by the brain and those produced by the ovaries, which have multiple and complex effects and relationships.

During premenopause and the reproductive years, cyclical interactions and cross-talk between the hormonal systems of the brain and the ovaries give rise to the monthly changes experienced by people who menstruate (see Box 2.1). This cross-talk between the brain and ovaries, and the typical cycle of hormones also drives the reproductive process, determining when in the month people might be able to conceive, with its fluctuations in estrogen and progesterone.

Box 2.1 A look at sex hormone fluctuation during premenopause and the reproductive years

In the brain, a hormone known as gonadotropin-releasing hormone (GnRH) stimulates production of two other hormones – luteinizing hormone (LH) and follicle stimulating hormone (FSH). These signal to the ovaries to produce the sex hormones estrogen and progesterone.[23] During the monthly cycle, estrogen and progesterone rise and fall in a cycle or pattern lasting approximately one month or 28 days (variable between individuals). This cycle is best envisaged as menstruation or a period (bleeding) happening at the beginning of the process, followed by ovulation at mid-cycle (at the end of what is referred to as the follicular phase) allowing for the possibility of fertilization, then a second phase (known as the luteal phase) that returns to the start of the cycle if fertilization does not occur.[24] In fact, as Figure 2.2 illustrates, in this monthly hormonal pattern, following menstruation, during the follicular phase, there is a dramatic peak in estrogen which then falls, signalling ovulation to begin; then in the luteal phase there's a steep rise in estrogen and progesterone followed by a dramatic drop, which signals bleeding and the cycle to begin again.

Follicular phase	Luteal phase

Estrogen (estradiol)

Progesterone

Period/menstruation

Ovulation

Hormone level

Beginning of cycle　　　　Mid-cycle　　　　End of cycle

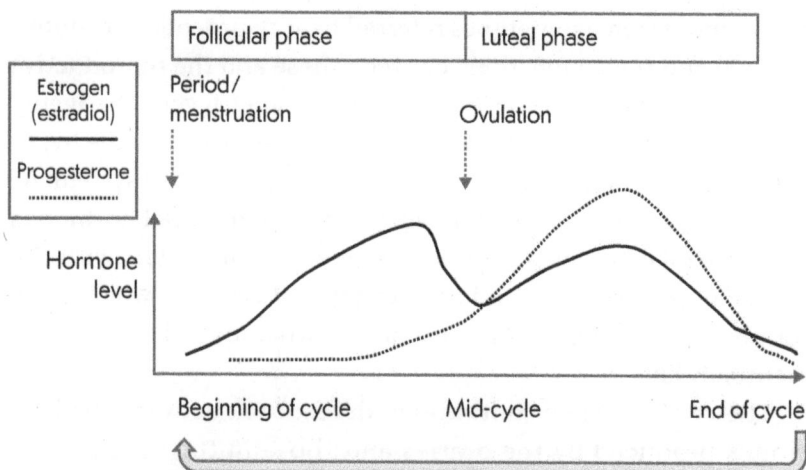

Figure 2.2 *Typical fluctuations in estrogen (estradiol) and progesterone hormones during the monthly menstrual cycle*

Estrogen and progesterone are involved in so much more than just ovulation and reproduction.[25] They are vital for maintaining a normal equilibrium in brain chemicals vital for mood and cognition, like serotonin and GABA. Monthly fluctuations in estrogen and progesterone have a particularly profound impact on emotion. Women and people assigned female at birth generally feel better at higher levels of estrogen, which occur mid-cycle, when they are in their 'fertile' phase, while we feel more anxious and depressed at lower levels, when progesterone dominates, later in the monthly cycle.[26] Progesterone, like estrogen, has substantive effects on mood, and as it decreases in the days before bleeding begins (towards the end of the luteal phase), we tend to feel more irritable, depressed and anxious.[27] This explains why people assigned female at birth are, sadly, at a higher risk of suicide during the late luteal and follicular phases (just before and during a period), since this is when estrogen and progesterone are at their lowest.[28] We will come back to this later, in Chapter 7, page 74: autistic people already struggle with their mental health, so hormonal fluctuations might be of even greater concern.

During menopause, the pattern of this cyclical hormonal dance starts to change, and communication between the two systems becomes increasingly out of sync. The changes that happen during the menopausal transition are due to interactions between the body's nervous system, including the brain, and hormonal or endocrine system (sometimes referred to as neuroendocrine inter-actions) and the connections between these and the reproductive processes in the ovaries. Hormone changes are triggered by ageing of parts of the brain involved in these processes (such as the hypo-thalamus) and ageing of the ovaries in the reproductive system. As the hypothalamus in the brain ages, some higher-level hormones that control estrogen and progesterone get out of sync with the usual monthly pattern. This has an effect on the ovaries, which when coupled with ovarian ageing, means that ovulation is disrupted and eventually fails.[29]

The cyclical dance continues with feedback between the hor-mones produced by the ovaries and those in the brain, but it becomes increasingly less graceful, or indeed dysregulated, over the menopausal process. Importantly, due to the dysregulation of hormones at the level of the brain, the pattern of decline in estrogen (specifically estradiol) produced from the ovaries becomes erratic; it doesn't just slowly decline from the start of perimenopause to postmenopause but repeatedly peaks and troughs as it falls over time, before declining more steadily after the final menstrual period and reaching a low point towards late postmenopause.[30] The sex hormone progesterone also decreases during perimenopause but at a slower and steadier rate until dropping to a low level in postmenopause.[31] This is why periods become irregular or erratic during perimenopause and eventually cease altogether. Similarly, in postmenopause, estrogen, progesterone and other reproductive hormones remain low, and without their regulatory hormones to suppress them, those hormones such as FSH and LH remain high[32] – it's as if the brain's hormonal system continues to prod that now unresponsive dance partner for the chemicals it's missing.

We've used the metaphor of a hormonal dance, but when we come to consider the experience of menopause and its symptoms, some might wonder what type of dance we are referring to: for many people it's more like a rollercoaster ride in respect to the symptoms they experience while these hormonal changes are happening. With this in mind, we move on to consider their physical impact on bodily symptoms and psychological impact on the person, in other words how 'the change' affects both body and mind, in the next chapter.

Chapter 3

'The change' and how it affects body and mind

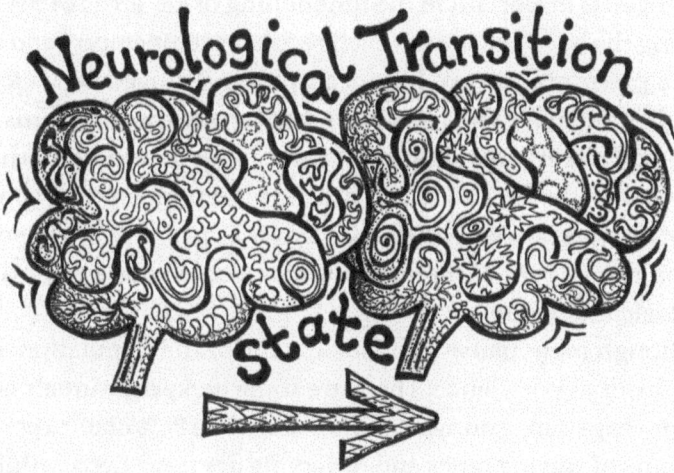

The neurological transition state that is menopause

When people think of menopause, they naturally tend to think of the ovaries and the reproductive system. However, the symptoms associated with menopause are actually largely neurological, at least in origin, and born of the interactions between the brain and other bodily systems.

Given the hormonal changes and dysregulation that are happening during menopause, multiple systems of the body become disrupted. The brain becomes less able to tolerate or make use of glucose (from the carbohydrates and sugars we consume) for metabolism and energy, and has to find other routes to accommodate this and regulate its energy,[1] resulting in a wide range of symptoms and impacts on health (as we'll discuss in Chapter 5). Changes in estrogen (specifically the type of estrogen called estradiol), in interaction with the hormones we've described, are responsible for the majority of symptoms experienced during menopause. Perimenopause, like puberty, is a neurological transition state – a time during which brain regulatory systems are restructured, and the brain moves from one developmental stage to another, where it's forced to function differently. While the extent and impact of the symptoms are often unexpected, they come as no surprise when considering the monumental changes happening in the brain, and the way the brain regulates and maintains many aspects of bodily functioning.

Estrogen is important in the functioning of key areas of the brain including the hypothalamus, which regulates temperature and sleep, and the prefrontal cortex, hippocampus and amygdala, which are involved in memory and learning[2] – hence why these systems get a bit 'wonky' during menopause. It's not just something hormonal happening in the ovaries, but it involves the brain and its complex array of interactions with the body. This is a crucial point when considering the impact of menopause for people with a pre-existing neurological difference.

Although menopause happens to 50% of the population, it is a very individual experience. There are some lucky individuals (about 20%) who experience no symptoms at all, while 80% of us experience symptoms of varying types and to varying degrees.[3] Even within one individual's menopause, their symptoms can be unpredictable and inconsistent: they might feel relatively 'normal' one day and experience a whole host of symptoms the next. Symptoms are known to be complex and diverse, and yet there are commonalities and universal experiences, which we'll explore here. To begin with, let's take a closer look at the cornucopia of symptoms that people can and may experience during menopause.

What are the symptoms of menopause?

There are many different symptoms associated with menopause: indeed, in one online survey, women aged 40 years and over identified an impressive 52 different symptoms, the top ones experienced being mood swings and brain fog.[4] There are also different ways of categorizing menopausal symptoms, such as physical, psychological, or a combination of both. In Figure 3.1, we have illustrated some of the types of symptoms associated with menopause, drawing on the argument that many menopausal symptoms are in fact neurological.[5] The wide range of menopause-related symptoms includes neurological effects such as vasomotor symptoms, cognitive dysfunction, changes in mood and emotion, sleep disruption and having headaches and migraines (Figure 3.1 top line), as well as other more wide-ranging symptoms such as cardiovascular and metabolic symptoms, joint and muscle pain, genitourinary symptoms such as vaginal dryness and exacerbation or flare-up of chronic conditions (Figure 3.1 lower line).

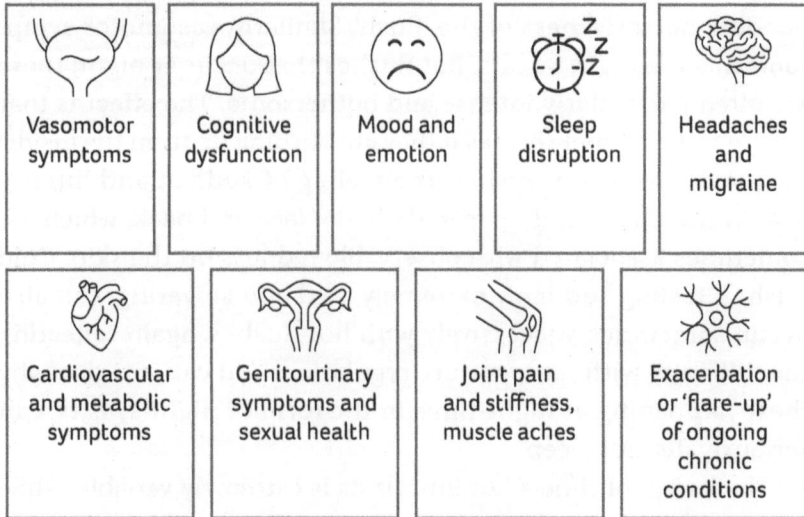

Vasomotor symptoms	Cognitive dysfunction	Mood and emotion	Sleep disruption	Headaches and migraine
Cardiovascular and metabolic symptoms	Genitourinary symptoms and sexual health	Joint pain and stiffness, muscle aches	Exacerbation or 'flare-up' of ongoing chronic conditions	

Figure 3.1 Types of symptoms associated with menopause

It's worth bearing in mind that there are differences of opinion between healthcare professionals about which symptoms are directly related to menopause and which might be related more to midlife ageing. Having reviewed a large proportion of menopause research, we suggest that the symptoms we discuss here are those associated with menopause and the menopausal transition, and into postmenopause, as we'll go on to explain.

Neurological symptoms: Vasomotor symptoms

Vasomotor symptoms, among the most stereotypical and classic signs of menopause, are caused by a disruption in the body's ability to control its temperature, resulting in the body's internal 'cooling down' signals being overexaggerated.[6] When this happens, the blood vessels dilate and the body sweats in an attempt to reduce the extreme heat it perceives there to be – rather like switching on full air conditioning when the winter sun only just starts to peep over the horizon. In menopause, this miscommunication in temperature signalling is caused by the fluctuations happening in sex hormones such as estrogen.[7] Vasomotor symptoms are more commonly known as hot flushes (or hot flashes, to use the US term). Interestingly, both terms refer to different qualities of this symptom: the suddenness of its onset in the 'flash' and the creeping, flooding pervasiveness of the 'flush'. Similarly, vasomotor symptoms include night sweats, hot flushes that occur at night; these are often particularly intense and bothersome. The effect is that people feel extremely hot, as if they are burning up from the inside; people describe hot flushes as a feeling of sudden and intense heat in the upper body, particularly the face and neck, which are sometimes associated with observable redness on the skin. Cold flushes, feeling suddenly extremely cold and shivering, can also occur, sometimes successively with hot flushes, again reflecting the difficulty with temperature regulation. You can imagine why these happening at night-time, in the form of night sweats, can seriously disrupt sleep.

The length of time a hot flush lasts is extremely variable: while most last seconds to minutes, some people report longer flushes lasting up to 60 minutes.[8] Hot flushes can also occur from a few to many times over the day and night, with some people reporting up to 50 of them over a period of 24 hours.[9] Even within the same person, vasomotor symptoms can vary considerably in frequency and intensity over time. Consequently, they range from being a minor irritation to severe and debilitating. In these more severe instances, hot flushes can create a sense of panic and fear of passing out; people may feel overwhelmed or as if they are 'going to burst with the heat'.[10] As an autistic participant in one of our studies put it:

" '... the sweats, I mean my whole body can get really hot... it's like an oven, and it is kind of embarrassing, going out... [it's] not only around my body but my back, it's just like drenched with sweat... the sweat, because it's so, so, the hot flush really kind of boils...'[11]

These feelings and symptoms can understandably have considerable impact on daily life, work and relationships. Vasomotor symptoms are reported to be the predominant symptoms of menopause for most people, and while they occur throughout the menopausal transition, they are particularly prevalent in late perimenopause and early postmenopause.[12] Data from one large-scale US study, appropriately named the SWAN study (Study of Women's Health Across the Nation), found that over the menopausal transition, vasomotor symptoms last on average for 7.4 years, with 4.5 years of this time actually during postmenopause.[13] Of the 80% of people who experience menopause symptoms, about a third experience only hot flushes, and the remainder have hot flushes in addition to a combination of other symptoms.[14]

Interestingly, vasomotor symptoms don't emerge in a uniform way across people of all countries, cultures and life circumstances. They're experienced by between 30% and 75% of women in low-income countries, but women in Asian countries rate them as less important than other types of menopausal symptoms.[15] We have already mentioned several sociodemographic factors that can influence the timing and experience of menopause symptoms, such as culture and ethnicity, age and educational level. In the SWAN study conducted in the USA, more African American women compared to white women reported having vasomotor symptoms[16] and they experienced these symptoms for longer than any other ethnic group examined, lasting on average over ten years.[17] Having a lower level of education has been identified as a risk factor for having worse vasomotor symptoms in late perimenopause and to a lesser extent in postmenopause, across almost all ethnic groups examined.[18] Also, having a history of more difficult premenstrual symptoms was associated with more severe vasomotor symptoms in the menopausal transition, particularly for white and Japanese women compared to other ethnic groups.[19] These sociodemographic differences might appear curious, and we'll come back to them in the chapters ahead, where we'll explain the underlying reasons for these disparities and their relevance to autistic people.

Neurological symptoms: Cognitive dysfunction, mood and emotion, sleep, headaches and migraine

Other menopause symptoms referred to as neurological often show up as what may also be thought of as psychological symptoms.[20] These symptoms include problems with memory (e.g. learning new things) and executive functioning (your ability to plan and adapt to the environment, control your attention, start and finish tasks, or switch between tasks). Thankfully, they appear to be largely temporary and many of them resolve at least to a degree in postmenopause,[21] but they can be intense and very difficult to live with while they last. Executive functioning difficulties are commonly referred to as **brain fog**, the feeling of being unable to think clearly, recall words or communicate fast enough, aptly described as feeling like you have 'a head full of cotton wool'.[22]

Similarly, symptoms related to mood and emotions include mood swings, and feelings of depression and anxiety, particularly in late perimenopause and postmenopause.[23] Depressive symptoms and diagnosed depression are more common in perimenopause and postmenopause than in the premenopausal years.[24] Increased anxiety, too, is a common symptom seen in the menopausal transition, regardless of whether anxiety was experienced before entering perimenopause.[25] Unfortunately for those who struggle with these emotional symptoms, both anxious and depressive symptoms, during menopause, have been linked to more severe and/or longer-lasting vasomotor symptoms and somatic symptoms (e.g. palpitations, headaches, feeling nauseous);[26] premenopausal anxiety has also been linked to a higher risk of vasomotor symptoms during the menopausal transition.[27]

Sleep disruption is another key neurological feature of menopause. It can manifest in a variety of ways, including difficulties falling asleep, night-time waking, awaking earlier than planned in the morning, feeling sleepy in the day, and the development of sleep disorders.[28] Headaches and migraine are common neurological symptoms during menopause, often causing severe pain and disruption in daily life and ability to work. One of our experts (Spike) referred to a particularly distressing 'combination of burnout and migraine'.

Other types of symptoms associated with menopause

Other symptoms in this challenging assortment include cardiovascular symptoms such as palpitations (being aware of the heart beating fast); pain from aching muscles and joints; and what are known as genitourinary (also called urogenital) symptoms, including increasingly irregular periods (which might come more or less frequently than expected during perimenopause), vaginal dryness, a decline in libido, urinary urgency or incontinence[29] and urinary tract infections. Finally, one lesser-known symptom is the worsening or flare-up of previously existing chronic health conditions, for example autoimmune diseases.[30]

Altogether, the impact of these symptoms can be formidable. Indeed, the physical and psychological effects of these symptoms can have an impact on a person's quality of life as well as that of their family, and invade every sphere of life, from personal to professional. They affect intimate relationships and sexual health,[31] and at an occupational level, have financial and economic impacts.[32] For example, a startling figure from a Fawcett Society report (2022) identified that one in ten women who were working at the time of menopause left their job because of menopausal symptoms.[33]

The complexity of menopause symptoms

Although it's possible to tease apart these individual symptoms and categorize them, as you saw above, they are highly interrelated and co-occur – especially the neurological symptoms.[34] Sleep difficulties seem to underlie the intensity of many of the menopausal symptoms, as you might imagine. For example, sleep disruption is frequently due to being woken several times each night by night sweats, particularly in late perimenopause and postmenopause;[35] the knock-on effects of not sleeping well appear to further intensify depressed mood and increased anxiety. There are many further symptoms beyond these associated with menopause, such as dry and itchy skin, including intensely itchy ears. In that long list of 52 symptoms we mentioned earlier,[36] other symptoms included tinnitus (ringing in the ears), dizziness and restless leg syndrome. Interestingly, the number of women reporting they had not experienced any of these 52 symptoms during menopause was zero.

The look and feel of menopause

Menopause also affects how your body looks and functions. People often find they gain weight during menopause, in part due to changes in metabolism, and they lose some of the agility that they were used to in their premenopausal years.[37] Both of these can be very hard to accept. This is relevant at menopause because it can affect some of the typical ways that people achieve a sense of self-worth. Sadly, it is very common for people to experience a loss of self-worth at menopause. These are comments from non-autistic women showing the impact of menopause on their sources of self-worth:

> 'I had to leave a well-paid position due to no support. I lost my house, my confidence and my self-worth. I felt like a failure.'[38]

> 'It didn't really stop my social life as such, but it definitely had an impact on relationships, on my self-worth. Feelings of not being worth – they were definitely really strong.'[39]

We have outlined the changes that occur at menopause, the range of physical, neurological and psychological symptoms that can be experienced as people transition through the menopausal process, and the impact that this can have across all dimensions of a person's quality of life. In the next chapter, we consider what factors might influence the way a person experiences menopause and the extent to which they experience symptoms. This is important to know for helping to reduce the impact of menopausal symptoms and in understanding why some people – like autistic people – may be particularly vulnerable to poorer health during menopause and beyond.

Chapter 4

The psychology of menopause

What factors can influence the way you experience menopause?

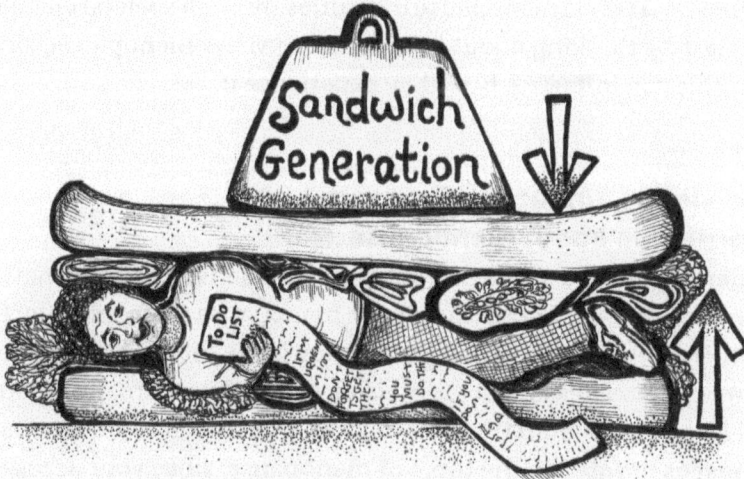

Put very simply, biological and hormonal factors are responsible for the phenomenon of menopause. However, there are a whole range of psychological, cognitive and emotional, social and cultural aspects which influence how a person experiences menopause, and that help to explain some of the differences experienced. We have already mentioned several sociodemographic factors (e.g. culture, ethnicity, age, educational level) and lifestyle factors (e.g. smoking, diet, exercise, BMI) that can influence the timing of menopause and experience of menopausal symptoms. But what about more individual psychological factors (e.g. the way we respond to emotions, the attitudes we hold, how we handle stress or the coping mechanisms we use), social influences (e.g. social relationships, family support, life circumstances, employment) and lifestyle factors (e.g. behaviours related to diet, exercise, sleep). How do these affect your experience of menopausal symptoms?

These are important to know, since most of the genetic and socio-demographic factors mentioned above may be pretty difficult or impossible to change. Although this is useful information in help-ing us to predict how a person might experience symptoms and identify who might be more vulnerable, and to focus support in the right direction, you can't do much individually to change some of these features. However, some personal psychological, social and lifestyle factors are able to be changed; others, if difficult to change for ourselves, highlight how important it is for those in positions of influence to tackle menopause inequities through societal changes. We start by thinking about how a person views menopause, since even this can influence how they experience it.

Knowledge, understanding and information about menopause

Evidence shows a wholesale and worldwide lack of information and consequently knowledge about menopause in people affected by it. There is a lot of variability in knowledge of menopause, both between countries and communities and within them. Knowledge and information aren't freely available, even when there are many webpages devoted to the topic of menopause, since your access to education affects your ability to find and understand these sources, as does your financial situation and employment status. This may be one reason why, as you saw in Chapter 3, page 37, having lower levels of education has been linked to more severe menopause symptoms.[1] People with lower educational attainment and lower socioeconomic status (those with less well-paid jobs, not in employment and/or living in poverty) tend, on average, to have less access to information and knowledge about menopause[2] – and people with less knowledge about menopause tend, on average, to have more severe symptoms.[3] This is also likely to be a factor in why African Americans, a group who, in the USA, have much poorer access to education and health-care, were found to have more severe symptoms.[4]

Where does lack of menopause information and education leave people? Well, it's not great. A lack of menopausal information and education can cause significant worry and concern for people entering perimenopause, encountering unexpected symptoms that they feel ill-prepared to deal with, and sending them on a convoluted, often frustrating journey to access healthcare and receive the answers, treatment, help and support they need. These sentiments were clearly expressed in the study we mentioned in the previous chapter, where women from the UK listed 52 different symptoms they had experienced since entering perimenopause.[5] Over 90% of these perimenopausal women reported not having been taught about menopause 'at all', and 60% felt they were not at all informed about it. In fact, when asked about perimenopause and menopause almost a third of them said they were 'dreading it' and most had only looked for information when they started to experience perimenopausal symptoms, usually from friends and websites. Bad enough that their personal knowledge and information was lacking, but these women were often frustrated when they sought advice and support from doctors and healthcare professionals.

We mentioned earlier that society as a whole is fairly uneducated about menopause,[6] and there's unfortunately also a lack of training and menopause education in healthcare professionals.[7] Women in this study were left feeling 'frustrated', 'annoyed', 'disempowered', 'confused' and 'unsupported'.[8] More broadly, they were upset and angry about the societal 'secrecy' surrounding perimenopause, which was treated as a 'hidden phenomenon'.[9] Participants in other studies have also observed a silencing of discourse around menopause and its symptoms, which comes with the tacit understanding that discussion should be minimized and symptoms privately endured.[10] This silencing harms people going through menopause, resulting in people not knowing what to expect and worrying that they are 'going mad' or developing early-onset dementia when deluged with menopausal symptoms.[11]

So, knowledge really is power, and people do better at menopause when they are well informed. Thankfully, public knowledge is slowly increasing with much greater visibility of menopause on social media and in celebrity accounts.[12] Although this does increase knowledge, information and understanding about menopause, it has had the unfortunate effect of centring the experiences and needs of white, cisgendered and middle-class women in heteronormative relationships.[13] It has also had the side effect of politicizing ageing, and medicalizing menopause as a deficiency or an illness in need of treatment.[14] We rarely hear about the positive aspects of menopause and while we wouldn't want to underplay the difficulties, recognizing positive experiences associated with menopause matters greatly. Knowing about positive aspects is important for transforming the image and stereotypes encountered by menopausal and postmenopausal people. This is why we've devoted a whole chapter to these later on (Chapter 18). Pathologizing menopause as something wholly negative that happens to people is not necessarily good for us[15] – we'll explain why in the following section.

Attitudes towards menopause and coping

Research from a range of studies worldwide has consistently shown that a person's attitude towards menopause influences their experience of symptoms. Specifically, having a more negative attitude towards menopause is associated with having more menopausal symptoms,[16] including hot flushes, night sweats, vaginal dryness, irritability, difficulty sleeping and headaches. There is at least some evidence that negative attitudes before menopause might be linked with more severe symptoms when it happens.[17] But let's pause for a moment, to think about the terminology that researchers use. Although not meant in this way, the phrase 'negative attitude' sounds a lot like having a bad attitude – a judgemental stance, which could be perceived as implying that symptoms are simply all in the mind, caused by the way a person thinks, or even seen as their own fault. To set the record straight, none of these things are true, far from it. We know there is an underlying biological cause of menopausal symptoms, but just as with any physical/bodily symptom, there are cognitive and emotional responses to symptoms influenced by personal, social and cultural factors, and your responses feed back into and affect your experience of the symptoms. While your cognitive and emotional responses to menopause are not your fault, if you're aware of the influence of your thinking style on your experience, it may be easier to tap into those cognitions and break the cycle.

Having a negative attitude towards menopause really refers to a person's expectations and beliefs about what menopause will be like to experience, and the impact that they envisage it will have on them personally, in their lives and their relationships with those around them. We prefer to think of this instead as 'menopause mindset', in just the same way as positive and negative mindsets have been applied to other things such as how stressful events are viewed.[18] Having a mindset that views the nature of the event or occurrence as debilitating (negative mindset) versus enhancing (positive mindset) can have very different physical and psychological effects, including on how symptoms are perceived and on quality of life.[19] We will see this later on in the accounts of our experts, and it's one reason why knowing about the positive aspects of menopause is important (Chapter 18).

When a person experiences physical or psychological symptoms of illness, they try to make sense of what is happening. They assess how dangerous the health symptoms are for them, how they will manage the symptoms, and what they need to do to deal with them in the future, drawing on cognitive resources including their own past experience of illness.[20] These mental processes produce illness cognitions or representations, which are essentially a person's beliefs about illness.[21] This way of understanding illness is grounded in a classic psychological theory of self-regulation, known as the Common-Sense Model.[22] It examines how someone labels the symptoms (identity), their beliefs about what causes them (cause), how long they are likely to last (timeline), the impact it might have (consequences), and if there is anything they can do to alleviate or stop the symptoms (cure). Why is this relevant? Well, while menopause is certainly not an illness, it is a condition with a range of symptoms, and this theory has very usefully been applied to the experience of menopause. Appraisal of symptoms associated with menopause has been referred to as cognitive menopausal representations.[23] To see what these might look like in reality, here are both positive and negative menopausal representations about the consequences of menopause, identified in a group of women in the UK:

" 'I had a few physical changes but nothing else; I'm still the same person.'[24]

❝ '... after my son was born I entered into a very rapid menopause... it started off with terrible night sweats. Waking up feeling very anxious. It was a horrible, horrible feeling... It was a loss of energy, self-respect, fears of getting old, being there for my youngest child. For the first time I had to face up to my own mortality...'[25]

While some research describes positive and negative menopausal representations as being similar across all stages of menopause, there is also evidence that postmenopausal people tend to have more positive cognitive and emotional representations of menopause.[26] Importantly, in relation to what we said earlier, these studies suggest that people with more negative representations of menopause tend to have a harder time during the transition. This is why having a very medicalized understanding of menopause as something bad that happens to you isn't necessarily helpful, and why researchers want to help people feel empowered during menopause, so that they feel more positive about it.[27]

Resilience factors linked with coping during menopause

Another way of framing psychosocial influences on menopausal symptoms and experience is thinking about protective or resilience factors (those that improve the experience and make it more positive), as opposed to vulnerability or risk factors (those that exacerbate the symptoms and lead to a more negative experience). Identifying resilience and vulnerability factors is a common goal in psychology and health research, and these are increasingly being examined and applied to menopause, to investigate what brings about the greatest chance of adaptation. Resilience factors that are effective during menopause have been found to include the degree of control a person feels they have over events in their life, having an optimistic outlook, a sense of purpose or meaning in life, and being aware of their emotions as well as how to regulate them effectively.[28] In a recent review, having one or more of these resilience and other resilience factors meant that a person was more able to adapt to menopause; this resulted in fewer and less severe menopausal symptoms (both physical and psychological), as well as having a better quality of life and improved wellbeing, and experiencing less perceived stress and fewer symptoms of depression.[29] We come back to some more about stress and control in Chapter 5.

Other research findings have pointed to both menopause-related and psychosocial risk and protective factors, specifically in respect to developing depression during menopause.[30] Interactions between already existing or ongoing vulnerabilities (e.g. having a history of depression before menopause, and a lot of stressful life events before or during menopause) and protective factors (e.g. having a positive menopausal attitude, treatment for menopause-related vasomotor symptoms, and receiving social support) can increase or decrease the risk of experiencing depression during menopause.[31] This shows that help is at hand and can be provided and tapped into in a variety of ways to improve the experience of menopause.

Menopausal challenges at midlife

To put menopause at midlife in context, we need to consider what else is happening at this mid-point in the lifespan: to broaden our lens to look at the psychological and social landscape of midlife, and most notably, the other challenges and ongoing life events people might be experiencing. Psychologists often talk about 'stressors', referring to things that people might perceive and experience as stressful in their lives. There's a lot going on during midlife. One large-scale survey in the USA found that wellbeing, including enjoyment and happiness, were at their lowest during ages 50–53 years in both women and men.[32] Compared to men, women scored lower on enjoyment but had similar levels of happiness. Though stress, anger and worry declined at midlife (and continued to reduce in older age), feelings of sadness were quite high in midlife – especially in women, who also had higher levels of stress, worry and sadness than men.[33] Though happiness and enjoyment increased again as people went into older age, this begs the question of why a midlife 'dip' in positive emotions happens.

Well, research in the general population suggests that midlife is a pivotal point in the lifespan, a time of both losses and of gains, and when the paradox of ageing is especially apparent.[34] Lachman and colleagues pointed out that declines in health and cognitive functioning (memory and executive functioning, such as planning and organizing your life) sit alongside, and are somewhat counterbalanced by, increases in knowledge and experience, and a greater ability to regulate emotions.[35] Whether this is also true for neurodivergent and autistic people, we are yet to find out. However, many neurodivergent people will be affected by the multiple acute and chronic stressors of midlife, which often occur at the same time or overlap in timing or duration. These stressors may be from different social domains of life, such as home, family and/or work, and people may experience them as utterly overwhelming, despite some of the coping tools they have acquired in their life so far. You might have heard of the term 'sandwich generation': Lachman and colleagues used this to describe the situational challenges of midlife.[36] It aptly explains the feeling of being placed in the middle of multiple demands and stressors, with demands from the generations above and below you, for example, having teenage children to care for at the same time as looking after ageing parents, or dealing with the demands of work, where you are junior to your manager but senior (and possibly responsible for) your junior colleagues. Unfortunately, we know that a lot of these pressures have a tendency to weigh more heavily on women and people assumed to be female.[37]

A key component of stress and what drives it is the concept of perceived control: the extent to which a person feels they are in control of and able to cope with the events they are experiencing.[38] Control is an important factor during midlife, since people can feel helpless in the face of the multiple co-occurring demands they are experiencing.[39] Alongside a lack of control, feeling that others are negatively judging you, a term referred as 'social evaluative threat', is also key to inducing and maintaining stress.[40] As Lachman and colleagues point out, despite multiple potential sources of stress, midlife also has multiple opportunities for feelings of accomplishment, satisfaction and mastery; hence the crossroads of midlife present a time when control is tested.[41] In people for whom control over events is particularly important, or who struggle with the social judgement of others, the stress of midlife might be even more overwhelming and present a time when they are tested in the extreme. This is highly relevant for autistic people, as we'll discuss in Part 2.

As you saw above, your menopause mindset, and how you cope with stress, can have considerable influence on how you experience menopause and the intensity of your symptoms. Feeling in control seems extremely important, in part because of how essential it is for coping with stress. People generally have an easier time at menopause when they feel they have some control over their menopausal symptoms and their overall health,[42] and they're more likely to feel in control if they're well educated and informed about menopause before it happens.[43] This may be partly why, as you'll come to see, neurodivergent people who don't understand what's happening to them often report feeling frightened and out of control during menopause (see Chapter 6, page 64, and Chapter 10, page 104), and why our experts advise other autistic people to learn as much as they can about menopause before (and when) it happens (Chapter 17, page 176).

You are not responsible for your attitude (your thoughts and feelings); we know how much these are shaped by your life experiences and innate temperament, as we'll discuss later in this book. However, this line of research is very appealing to psychologists because awareness and attitudes towards menopause are things we can change, often through psychological interventions.

This said, although your attitudes about menopause, stress and coping are important, we also need to grapple with the fact that the biological stress response undergoes changes during midlife and menopause. This may disadvantage women and people assigned female at birth when it comes to coping with menopausal and midlife stress. We know that during the menopausal transition, there is an increase in the underlying levels of the stress hormone cortisol, which appears to be linked to more severe vasomotor symptoms.[44] While earlier in life, men seem more reactive to stress than women, this pattern seems to reverse during menopause, such that by the time they are postmenopausal, women show a greater cortisol response to stressful challenges than do men of the same age and younger, premenopausal women.[45] These stress effects appear to be mediated by changes in estrogen and other menopause hormones.[46] This suggests that hormone changes that happen during the menopausal transition may create a heightened vulnerability to stress, which ironically might further exacerbate menopausal symptoms.[47]

Stress is a large part of why we think menopause might be especially challenging for neurodivergent people, so we need to spend some time understanding it. In the next chapter, we take a closer look at stress, both stressful events that occurred in the past and ongoing stressors in the present. We think about how it can affect a person's health during menopause, as well as beyond in the years ahead.

Chapter 5

Why does menopause matter?

Relationships between menopause and health

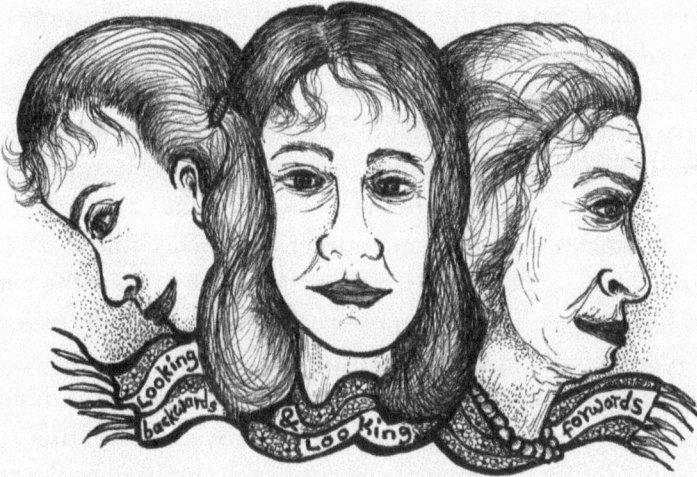

Menopause certainly does matter; it matters for health in the here and now, during the menopausal transition, but it also matters for future health across the lifespan. This is because health during menopause has implications for health later in life as people age, setting the scene for future struggles or future protective effects. The experience of stress and how people respond to life's challenges, as we've already suggested, have rather a large part to play in all this. We begin this chapter by explaining what we mean by stress and describe what happens to our biology and psychology when we face challenging or threatening situations and experiences.

The biology of stress

In Chapter 4, we pointed out that the combination of menopause and midlife stress can create a situation of potential vulnerability for people going through menopause, at both a biological and psychological level. In fact, stress can have a considerable impact on health by altering physical functioning across the whole range of bodily systems, since the consequences of stress and trauma are not just 'in the mind'; they are physically written on the body and brain.

The biological stress response is actually a good way of dealing with challenges – it automatically enables us to fight, flee, freeze or fawn in the presence of a threat. This stress response evolved to keep us safe against predators, intended as a short-lived or acute response to get us out of danger.[1] But when the stress response becomes prolonged over time, when multiple or complex stressors are drawn out over months or years, particularly when stress is due to ongoing negative or threatening social interactions, the chronic stress we experience can physically change the brain and have harmful effects on the body.[2] Those changes to the brain also make us more sensitive to subsequent stress that we encounter, and we become more easily triggered when we confront stress in the future. It's like the person is on a hair-trigger: they can more easily go from 0 to 60 miles per hour in terms of responding strongly and quickly to things that might not have affected them so severely in the past. This might be adaptive when you're living in a jungle where you encounter tigers every other day but is less adaptive when your brain rings the alarm bells for a wide range of social threats from which you can't escape.

Chronic (long-lasting) stress impacts every organ system in the body, including the cardiovascular, neuroendocrine and immune systems, making us more vulnerable to serious illness. Stress we experience in the here and now, during midlife and the menopausal transition, can have effects on future health. However, stress we experienced in the past, prior to midlife, can also be carried forwards. Menopause presents itself at that crossroads where the stress of your previous years catches up with you, manifesting as you go through this biological transition and the accompanying multiple stressors of midlife, and possibly making ripples that will affect you in the future.

Past stress showing up in the present

What kind of life experiences are scored into the body and mind when a person enters midlife? Studies have shown that stress experienced due to early life adversity or adverse childhood experiences (e.g. emotional, physical or sexual abuse, neglect or family dysfunction during childhood) can have physical effects on the body that emerge during midlife and into older age. However, it's not only childhood stress that can have an effect at midlife. Chronic stress during adulthood (e.g. due to stressful life events such as poverty, employment difficulties, bereavement, physical assault, relationship breakdown, and everyday and major incidents of discrimination) have been linked to poorer physical health in midlife.[3] In fact, the stress and trauma of childhood and adulthood, both separately and combined, have been found to accelerate biological ageing in middle-aged people, with childhood stress particularly associated with ageing in women.[4] To have accelerated biological ageing means that the body shows more signs of wear and tear and poorer health (including illnesses of older age) than you would expect in people of that age. Accelerated ageing due to stress and trauma can even be associated with earlier death.[5] This is particularly pertinent when you consider the lower life expectancy of autistic people.[6] It's really important to emphasize here that not all individuals with lifetime trauma will die younger. It's only when we look across large numbers of people, in science, that we see these trends.

When it comes to natural menopause in adulthood, happening during midlife, the health consequences of this accumulation of life's stress and trauma are highly relevant. This may be why people with a history of prolonged stress and trauma, whose bodies may have aged faster than their peers, enter menopause slightly earlier, on average.[7] Earlier age at natural menopause is generally not a good thing – it means that your body spends more time in a state of estrogen deprivation, and so is associated with more negative health consequences, and even earlier death.[8]

A history of life stress not only influences when you enter menopause, but how you experience it. It seems that when estrogen declines at menopause, the impacts of stress and trauma on the brain are unmasked, becoming more evident.[9] This means that menopausal people with a history of stress tend to have more severe menopausal symptoms, including vasomotor symptoms and emotional and cognitive change.[10] In two studies of menopausal women, adverse childhood experiences were found to have had a negative impact on the brain network responsible for executive functioning, and impairments emerged strongly as the neuroprotective effect of estrogen dwindled.[11] Impacts of earlier life stress emerged in other ways, too. Data from the SWAN study in menopausal American women showed that the chronic social stress of everyday discrimination was associated with increases in inflammatory markers and higher blood pressure,[12] which indicate a greater vulnerability for developing cardiovascular disease in the future. If you remember back to Chapter 3 (page 37), the same SWAN study reported more severe and enduring vasomotor symptoms in African American participants particularly[13] – it's almost certain that prolonged experiences of minority stress and discrimination have something to do with this. Being aware of such experiences and vulnerabilities and how they might show themselves at menopause can help people's needs to be understood, and can assist with providing and receiving the most appropriate intervention and support (more about this in Part 4).

Social support offers protection

There are things that can protect us from the harmful impacts of stress, and it's worth thinking about these because autistic people may have them in lesser amounts, if at all. Psychologists are very interested in social relationships and the social support we receive from other people, as well as the support we are able to give to others. Sources of social support can be from a person's partner, family and friends, as well as formal sources including healthcare providers. There are different ways to describe the many types of social support, but these can include tangible help (e.g. having someone who will bring you your shopping or give you a lift to a medical appointment), belonging support (e.g. having people to do things with, who make you feel connected and part of a social circle), self-esteem support (e.g. having someone who compliments you, makes you feel good about yourself), and appraisal support (e.g. having someone with whom you can weigh up your situation, who can help you feel more positive about a situation and your ability to cope).[14] All of these forms of social support can protect people, to some extent, from the negative impacts of stress, and are linked with better health and wellbeing.[15]

Given the stressful challenges we've already talked about, menopause is a time where people might be especially in need of support from others. Being in receipt of social support has been found to promote more positive attitudes towards menopause, which, as we heard in Chapter 4, has the beneficial effect of reducing symptoms experienced.[16] We can see this in accounts from non-autistic people, who in one study of mainly British white women, spoke about a 'menopause sisterhood' among cisgender women who share the same kinds of difficult experiences.[17] Indeed, many of the women in this study expressed that the empathy, validation and non-judgemental support they received from other women was more helpful than the support they received from male partners.[18]

There also exists a more unhelpful or negative side to social support, which may be particularly relevant to experiences during menopause and those menopausal experiences of neurodivergent people. Interestingly, not all studies have found social support to improve vasomotor symptoms, possibly because some types of support, such as discussing symptoms, might for some people have the effect of making them more aware of what they might experience and set up negative expectations.[19] Similarly, the positive solidarity expressed in the menopause sisterhood study described above was not felt by cisgender women whose menopause was different in some way (e.g. those with different symptoms, or who had a premature or medical menopause).[20] Instead, they found that this difference left them outside of the circle of 'solidarity', with their friendship group having 'broken down' and feeling 'less connected'.[21] So where menopause didn't fit the usual expectations in symptoms or timing, seemingly supportive social relationships actually contributed to negative feelings of stress.[22] It follows that anyone experiencing a different kind of menopause, perhaps as a transgender man or indeed as a neurodivergent person, might find themselves similarly out in the cold within existing friendships.

Lack of positive support can have negative consequences for health, and support from healthcare providers has also been found lacking during menopause. In a recent UK study, almost 20% of people who visited a healthcare practitioner in search of help or support during menopause reported that they received none, and this was particularly the case for those in early perimenopause.[23] Women who had been through a medically induced menopause also reported being less satisfied with the healthcare they had received compared to women in late perimenopause.[24] A common theme in this study was of people feeling dismissed rather than supported by their healthcare providers, in some cases being told directly that support was not needed for people going through menopause:

> " '... menopause is a natural process that the majority of women go through with no need for support...'[25]

This attitude seems even more misguided when we consider what we know about the impact of menopause on mental and physical health more broadly. Helping people manage or even optimize their health and wellbeing during menopause is imperative for their future, as we'll go on to discuss.

Health during menopause and future health

If you've been following our discussion so far, you'll see that in the melting pot of health during menopause, there are the long-term effects of earlier life adversity or stress, wear and tear on the body and brain that may manifest clearly during midlife, exaggerated by menopausal changes. There are the neurological changes associated with the menopausal transition and the mental health vulnerabilities they can induce, as we discussed in Chapters 2 and 3, and there are also a wide range of effects across the rest of the body. Menopausal changes can influence a range of biological systems, including those that usually sustain cardiovascular and immune functioning, and enable bone health and metabolic changes.[26] This means that menopause can worsen physical illnesses or disabilities, or it can introduce new ones. As such, the perimenopausal period is seen as a time of greater vulnerability, with increased risk for a number of mental and physical health conditions.[27] For this reason, experts suggest that the stage of perimenopause may be a critical or sensitive period of the lifespan, determining future health in older age, and even life expectancy.[28]

We touched on mental health and mood disorders in Chapter 2 (page 31) and Chapter 3 (page 38) – it will come as no surprise to anyone who's been through it, but menopause can really affect a person's mental health, regardless of their neurotype. Though anxiety and low mood are quite common menopausal symptoms, there is some evidence that menopause may be a particularly vulnerable time for the onset or recurrence of mental illnesses like depression, schizophrenia and bipolar disorder.[29] This is most likely due to an interaction between the sex hormone alterations of menopause and disruption of the stress response.[30] Unfortunately, as you saw in Chapter 2, declining estrogen disrupts brain chemicals, like serotonin and GABA, which are strongly implicated in mental illness.[31] Some non-autistic people describe developing debilitating anxiety and intense depression during menopause,[32] problems which are worsened by sleep disturbance. For some people, things get so bad that they feel life is no longer worth living, as indicated in these comments from neurotypical women:

" 'I feel desperate... I have been frighteningly close to walking into traffic so I can end my life.'[33]

" 'I realized the depression anxiety was getting worse and worse... I was just a shell; I'd drag myself around.'[34]

On a grand scale, the link between mental illness, suicide and menopause may also be reflected in UK-wide statistics: in 2022, deaths by suicide were more common in women aged 45–64 than any other female age group, although these could not be specifically linked to menopause.[35] The relationship between menopausal hormone changes and suicide isn't straightforward; some studies find higher prevalence of suicidal thoughts in perimenopausal and postmenopausal people, but not all do.[36] For those who go into menopause with pre-existing mental illnesses, though, any further deterioration in their mental health is a serious threat, given the heightened suicide risk associated with mental illness.[37]

Other particularly heightened health risks during menopause

include autoimmune, cardiovascular and metabolic conditions. Existing or underlying autoimmune conditions appear to be worsened by changes in estrogen and other hormones, such that during menopause, people might experience the onset or worsening of conditions such as systemic lupus erythematosus, rheumatoid arthritis, type 1 diabetes and autoimmune thyroid disease.[38] In relation to metabolic and cardiovascular diseases, increased vulnerability seems to occur due to increases in the distribution of body fat, weight gain and greater insulin resistance; this results in the body being increasingly unable to break down glucose and increases in cholesterol.[39] Feeding forward into later life, cardiometabolic risk factors during menopause, like high blood pressure, have been found to be consistently associated with cardiovascular disease later on in post-menopause (average age 60 years).[40] Fascinatingly, this is another area where we can see the complex interplay between psychological factors, like how well supported you feel, and your physical health. Thinking about social support, mentioned above, research suggests that emotional expression within intimate partner relationships is important for cardiovascular health in midlife women.[41] In a study of women aged 40–60 years, those who self-silenced in their relationship (avoided expressing or asserting themselves in order to keep the peace) were more likely to show signs of developing cardiovascular disease in the arteries supplying blood to the brain.[42] Although self-silencing might not be quite the same as the kind of masking that autistic people do (see Chapter 9, page 90), the parallel is disquieting – both involve suppressing your true thoughts and feelings, which is stressful and tiring. Interestingly, some people find themselves less inclined to self-silence – or indeed to mask – during the menopausal transition, as we'll come back to in Chapter 15 (page 157). Some of our autistic experts described this as a positive aspect of menopause (Chapter 18, page 184).

While these conditions are highlighted as a particular risk during menopause, the impacts of menopause throughout the body are so widespread and so great that it would be hard to list them all. Little attention is paid to chronic illnesses and physical disabilities during this time, but they stand to be affected in ways that many people might take for granted. Given the neuroprotective effect of estrogen, menopause can worsen the symptoms of conditions affecting the brain and nervous system, like multiple sclerosis, fibromyalgia and chronic fatigue syndrome/myalgic encephalomyelitis (CFS/ME).[43] Declining estrogen makes skin thinner and more fragile, which can make people with reduced mobility even more vulnerable to skin tears and pressure sores.[44]

So, menopause at midlife is where many roads meet. A time where, thinking back to the previous chapter, we are exposed to a landscape of midlife stressors, which we're more sensitive to due to the biological changes occurring. A time where present stress actually takes a more severe toll on our health, where past stress makes itself known, and where our bodies can take on additional wear and tear, affecting future health. It really is the crossroads at the midpoint of life – the past manifesting in the present, forming a pathway, albeit frequently traversed via a rollercoaster ride, from premenopausal to postmenopausal life. It couldn't be more important that people are supported during this time. Although we've highlighted some of the health risks that people can face during menopause, the fact that it's a sensitive period, a crossroads in life,[45] also makes it an opportunity for intervention to improve subsequent health across the lifespan, as we'll discuss later in this book.

In the first part of this book, we've hopefully set the scene, discussing both the biology and psychology of the menopausal experience and the crucial interaction between them, focusing on the important links between menopause and health more generally. You've seen the many ways that a person's menopausal experience can differ, and some of the reasons why. It's against this backdrop that we go on to consider why this journey might present particular difficulties for autistic people and those who are neurodivergent.

Part 2

AUTISTIC AND MENOPAUSAL: THE 'DOUBLE WHAMMY'

In this second part, we'll delve deeper into why menopause might be particularly challenging for autistic people, gathering the threads we introduced in Part 1 and examining them through an autistic lens. When people call something 'a double whammy', they usually mean that a person is being 'slammed' by two challenging situations at once. We use it here because some autistic people we've spoken to suggest that the combination of these two things, being autistic and being menopausal, brings additional challenges over and above those associated with either of them alone. Indeed, some autistic people speak of 'autistic menopause':[1] a term which suggests unique aspects of the autistic menopausal experience.

You might have started to guess some of the reasons why autistic people might struggle during menopause – we'll summarize them in Chapter 7 before going into more detail in the following chapters. In particular, we reconsider the midlife landscape discussed in Chapter 4 and think about the midlife terrain autistic people might face (Chapter 8). Having considered the importance of how we feel and think about menopause, we discuss the importance of knowing about autistic menopause and autism itself (Chapter 9). We'll also consider the additional challenges that might come with different forms of neurodivergence (Chapter 10), and other kinds of marginalized identity (Chapter 11). First, Chapter 6 starts with our experts and their thoughts on what menopause means to them.

Chapter 6

Autistic experts

'If I could use one word to describe my experience of menopause'

66 *'Challenging.'* SPIKE

66 *'Confusing.* I find it very difficult to know what is related to menopause and what isn't.' ALICE

66 *'Crazy.* A crazy world I was living in all of a sudden. Everything sort of... went from being what I had known to being something completely different. I started to feel completely overwhelmed and I couldn't understand.' BRIDIE

66 *'Enlightening*... I learnt a lot... the one thing women have in common... is that we're going to go through it... it has a huge effect on your entire way of being.' THE CAT

66 *'Sweat!* I never used to perspire. Now it's like a tap, basically!' BASSAI SHO

66 *'Change*... just so many changes that I went through during the menopause and the life before and after.' CLAIRE

66 *'Traumatic.* My hormones were all over the place. My emotions were too. I couldn't think straight. I was in pain, so much pain.' FLORENCE

66 *'Anxiety.* It was one of the main things that led me to realize that I was

going through the menopause. One of the biggest, biggest differences was my anxiety became... debilitating.' JANET

" '**Bloody**. I once gave a presentation to a bunch of mostly male staff. I entitled it "Blood Sweat and Tears".' SALLY

" '**Nightmare**... I thought I was losing my mind.' ANNE

" '**Hell**... it totally turned my life upside down.' DAISY

" '**Confused**. I really can't articulate what is the menopause, what is burn-out, what is just getting older... it's so difficult to parse what's happening.' TARA

" '**Bewildering**; overwhelming, awful. There was so much emotion going on and sleep [problems]... it magnified everything.' KATIE

" '**Confusing**. You get used to being in your own body to a degree, and then all this other stuff starts happening... I've got synaesthesia, so my senses get mixed up and I get sensory overload as well. When stuff starts happening in your body, you're... hyper-aware of it.' SUZI

" '**Soul-destroying**. You kind of have an idea what you think [menopause] might consist of and you think that you're prepared, but when it actually happens to you... it literally has changed everything about who I am. No matter how much I try to counteract the menopausal symptoms, there's something else I can't get around.' ANN

Our autistic experts came up with a wide range of words to describe their experiences of menopause. For Janet, Sally and Bassai Sho, certain symptoms like hot flushes, flooding and anxiety so affected them as to remain their lasting impression of menopause. Others (Daisy, The Cat) described an all-encompassing experience, hard to grasp and understand, which affected their whole lives. These words really capture the smorgasbord of symptoms that we talked about in Part 1, and particularly the neurological nature of menopause (page 33). Ann's comment, that it changed everything about them, reminds us that the brain is the seat of the mind, which gives rise to our conscious experiences and perceptions of the world. As such, it makes perfect sense that changes in the brain, as happen in menopause, can affect everything about the way we exist in and experience the world. Anne's comment about 'losing my mind' makes sense in this context: you're not losing it, but your mind is changing at menopause, so you might feel it in every corner of your life. Claire spoke about her life before and after menopause, and Bridie referred to life being 'completely different' afterwards.

Confusion and distress were two feelings that left a lasting impression on several of our experts. For Tara and Alice, it was hard to separate out symptoms of menopause from other things going on in their lives, such as burnout and stressful life experiences. Bridie and Katie spoke about feeling 'overwhelmed', being caught in the middle of this 'crazy world'; for Katie and for Florence too, emotions were 'magnified' and 'all over the place'. For Lily, being caught in this maelstrom was 'exhausting'; for Ann, there was a sense of being helpless to counteract the symptoms. Such confusion and distress are understandable, as this can indeed be a 'challenging' time, to use Spike's word. It can be hard enough to learn how to be in our bodies, as Suzi expressed, without them going and changing on us in a way we can't fully control.

Yet The Cat spoke about this time as 'enlightening'. They didn't choose to experience it as they did, but as we continue through this book, we will see that each of our experts grew through this time, gaining hard-won knowledge. In fact, menopause does not need to have a negative meaning; it should not need to be 'traumatic' (Florence). As we saw in Chapter 4, people across the world think about it in very different ways.[1] Interestingly, some cultures think about and experience menopause as a liberating experience, granting freedom from dietary, social and religious restrictions associated with menstruation, and they honour the wisdom of menopausal women. In some cultures, menopause is marked only by periods stopping, and little by other symptoms.

Again, this is absolutely not to say that people are responsible for their menopause mindset and the way they experience menopause. It is just to acknowledge that culture has a lot to answer for. It seems to us that some of the suffering expressed by our autistic experts comes from their going into menopause unprepared and disempowered, some undiagnosed, in a culture that isn't set up to understand or support neurodivergent people at menopause. We hope this can change, and if we were to ask the same question to autistic people in ten years' time, we might get different answers.

Chapter 7

Why might menopause be harder for autistic people?

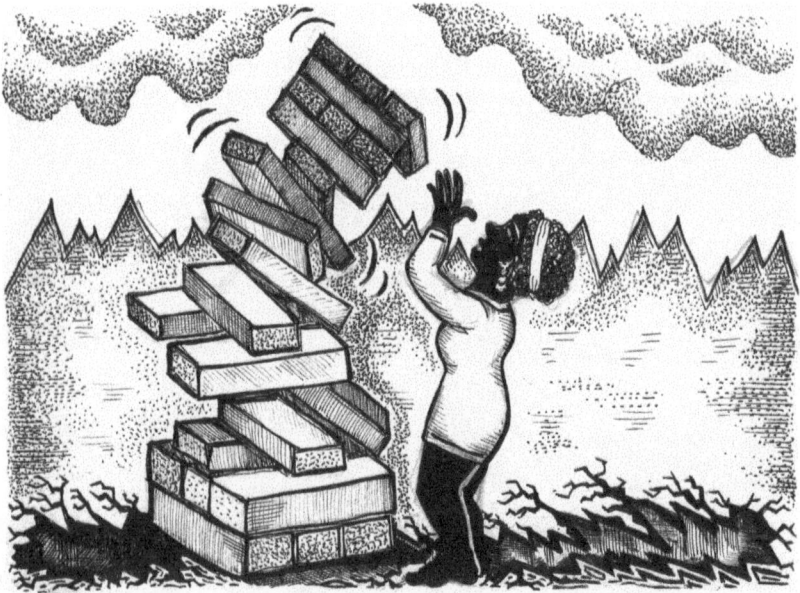

Not all autistic people will have a difficult time at menopause. As you've seen over the previous chapters, there's a huge deal of variation, with some non-autistic people having a very hard time; we've seen similar variation in our studies, with some autistic people reporting a relatively easy menopause. Yet there are a number of reasons why autistic people might be more likely to have a particularly difficult time during menopause. These reasons fall into autism-related factors, those that are related to general aspects of health and wellbeing, and those that are related to the environment and life experiences common to autistic people (see Figure 7.1). Some of these also affect other neurodivergent people, as we'll discuss in Chapter 10.

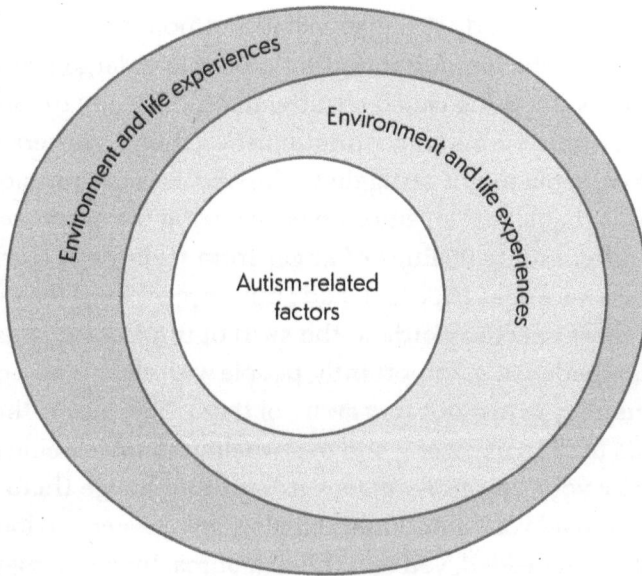

Figure 7.1 *Vulnerability factors that might affect autistic people at menopause*

Autism-related factors

Beginning with the innermost circle in Figure 7.1, we first consider autism-related factors as vulnerabilities at menopause.

Autistic people struggle with change, especially when it's unpredictable

Autistic people naturally struggle with change, uncertainty and unpredictability, all of which are a major source of anxiety.[1] Autistic people often like to deeply understand a topic, such as how the body works, and might want to understand their menopause symptoms at a precise and scientific level. Unfortunately, if you think back to those fluctuating hormones in Chapter 2, you can see why menopausal symptoms are fundamentally unpredictable. We don't have a window into our brains to understand what's happening at any given time, and even doctors cannot give us a personalized roadmap. Menopause cannot always be definitively diagnosed by medical tests, and as we've seen, doctors differ in their knowledge and opinions about it.[2] This is extremely difficult for those who struggle with unpredictability.

Autistic people already struggle with their emotions

Emotions are challenging for autistic people. A large proportion experience something called alexithymia: a difficulty understanding your own emotions and communicating them to others. People with alexithymia might struggle to differentiate the physiological sensations that signal an emotion is occurring (for instance, being able to differentiate feelings of anger from feelings of fear). They might be aware that they feel 'bad', but beyond that, they cannot pin any more specific words to the swirl of unpleasant sensations they are experiencing. Importantly, people with alexithymia do have emotions; they're just not very aware of them. This means that their emotions tend to be strong and overwhelming, since being unable to identify your emotions makes it hard to manage them. If you struggle to read your emotional signals and take steps to look after yourself when needed, you run the risk of reaching boiling point – or indeed, meltdown – where emotions explode out in uncontrolled and often embarrassing ways. Some resort to harmful behaviours such as self-harm,[3] disordered eating[4] or even suicide attempts,[5] as a way to manage or escape distressing emotions.

The new experience of powerful and unstable emotions at menopause is very distressing for non-autistic people,[6] and the broader life changes of midlife make it a time of potentially strong emotions. For autistic people who already struggle with emotions, any heightening of these problems may be very detrimental.

Autistic people already struggle with some cognitive processes

Cognitive processes like attention, planning and memory are often tricky for autistic people. Psychologists often think of attention like a spotlight which can be narrowed in to focus on one thing, or widened to illuminate many things in the environment. Usefully, most non-autistic people can more easily widen and focus that spotlight and move their attention from one thing to the next. For autistic people, it is like the spotlight of their attention is stuck on 'focus', and they can't shift it easily between different targets.

In some contexts, autistic attention can be a wonderful thing: autistic people are often very good at sustaining their attention over long periods, or focusing on fine-grained details. They can be immensely productive and achieve a deep sense of satisfaction and purpose in these states of hyper-focus or flow, even if they might forget to sleep or eat.[7] The problematic thing seems to be controlling their attention when it comes to moving from one task to another, or paying attention to numerous things at a shallower level. Dividing your attention across multiple targets is a necessity when multitasking, so it stands to reason that many autistic people struggle with this.

The ability to control your attention is an aspect of executive function, a major difficulty for autistic people (and ADHDers). Difficulties with executive function also show up difficulties making, adapting and carrying out a plan to achieve your goals, whether those are major goals (like finishing an assignment) or minor goals (making a cup of tea, which requires sequencing actions like getting the milk out of the fridge and boiling the kettle).[8] Autistic challenges with executive function also come up in the concept of autistic inertia, which is difficulty starting or stopping an action. Some autistic people describe it as the 'most disabling part of being autistic', affecting their self-worth, their relationships, education and employment.[9] Finally, while some autistic people have very good memories for things that happened in the longer-term past,[10] autistic people typically struggle with the aspect of memory which is linked to executive function[11] – the ability to hold information in your short-term memory so you can readily access it, which psychologists call working memory.

These things are hard enough, but many autistic people learn to live with them. However, as a neurological transition which affects these processes, menopause may be an additional load on cognitive processes that are already challenging. As we discussed in Chapter 3, menopausal symptoms are strongly interrelated, and cognition and emotion are closely intertwined. For example, studies from non-menopausal autistic people tell us that anxiety freezes up the engine of cognition, making executive function even more difficult.[12] As such, the strong emotions that are associated with menopause, which might well be amplified for autistic people, might make thought processes even more difficult.

Autistic people already struggle with their senses and their physical bodies

How humans experience the world is like a constant ongoing conversation between the brain and our environment, with the body (the senses) carrying messages between the two. Like many things in life, this conversation is a lot more complicated for neurodivergent people; these messages from the senses get transmitted too loudly, or not loudly enough. Autistic people often experience their senses differently to non-autistic people – whether that's sight, sound, smells, taste, touch and/or internal signals (also known as interoception). For those who are hypersensitive to light, sounds and smells, these things can be physically painful, sickening and 'utterly overwhelming'.[13] The sense of touch spans many things, from human contact to the feeling of wearing socks; it also affects eating, given the textures of different foods. Many autistic people will avoid certain places, people, materials and foods because of their hypersensitivity, which very much affects different parts of their lives.[14] Interestingly, it is possible to be over-sensitive to some senses but under-sensitive to others: as such, you'll also find some autistic people will seek out certain textures, feelings of pressure (e.g. weighted blankets), colours and strong flavours. The feeling of saying a word or making a sound, watching a repetitive motion, touching, smelling or tasting something, can bring immense joy and comfort.[15]

Interoception, our ability to notice and understand signals from our body (e.g. feelings of thirst, hunger, being full, too hot or too cold, feeling sick, needing the toilet), is also challenging for autistic people. Under-sensitivity to these kinds of bodily signals can be embarrassing, leading to accidents in the toileting department; at worst, it can be harmful, when autistic people do not realize they are ill or the severity of an injury.[16] Some autistic people may be acutely aware of the various odd things the body does, its squishes and gurgles, and get very anxious about these.

It is possible that some of the symptoms of menopause, such as hot flushes, might be especially troublesome for autistic people, given their existing sensitivity to the way they feel and the ways they experience the world through their senses. We don't know enough, yet, about how interoceptive differences in autistic people might affect them at menopause. Studies of the brain have shown that during hot flushes, there is activity in the parts of the brain involved in interoceptive awareness of temperature:[17] this is consistent with the anxious, uncomfortable thoughts that people experience during hot flushes.[18] We also know that in neurotypical people, heightened 'symptom sensitivity' – the degree to which people are aware of noises, temperature, hunger, pain and internal bodily functions – is related to longer duration of vasomotor symptoms.[19] It might be that for those autistic people who are very sensitive to and distressed by their bodily signals, hot flushes are even more overwhelming and anxiety-inducing. Feeling something 'happening' without being fully able to understand what is going on could be really unpleasant.[20] Indeed, qualitative work touching on the topics of autistic menopause and interoception suggests that the changes of menopause can be quite discombobulating for those with interoceptive differences.[21]

As we mentioned earlier, menopause also affects how your body looks and functions, something which can be difficult for both autistic and non-autistic people to accept. Interestingly, body acceptance and satisfaction, in autistic people, appears to be based not only on how the body looks, but how it feels and what it can do.[22] Knowing what to expect from your body (and how to take care of it) is extremely important for autistic people. With the changes of puberty, some autistic people describe feeling like their body no longer belongs to them.

Some autistic people living in bigger bodies are badly affected by societal stigma around weight and size, and experience negative self-image as 'a source of mental anguish throughout their lives'.[23] It is important to recognize that autistic people are more likely than non-autistic people to live with eating disorders,[24] conditions where the number on the scale, or their clothes size, affects their self-worth to an agonizing extent. These factors together mean that changes in the way your body works, feels and looks might be harder to navigate as an autistic person.

Health- and wellbeing-related factors

In the next layer of vulnerability factors (Figure 7.1), we consider health- and wellbeing-related vulnerabilities.

Autistic people already struggle with low self-worth

To say that this is a tough world to live in as an autistic person is something of an understatement! Autistic people often have to contend with school and workplace environments which are not adapted to them, where they will struggle to perform at their best.[25] Having a minority kind of brain, in a world where you are different from others, can make autistic people feel very broken and deficient. Being victimized and excluded by other people only adds to this.[26] It will come as no surprise that most studies find that autistic adults have pretty low self-esteem.

People with low self-esteem can be very vulnerable. Often, we affix our self-worth to something outside of ourselves, and pursue that thing in order to escape those awful feelings of badness, brokenness or failure.[27] With so many autistic people struggling with low self-worth, what kinds of goals do they reach for in order to feel better about themselves? Sometimes, they strive for self-worth by trying to change how their body looks or how much it weighs.[28] Sometimes, they get self-worth from how others treat them, how socially adept they feel,[29] or how sexually desirable. Sometimes it is from excelling in a sport, musical or creative pursuit; from being productive; progressing in their career; or doing well at school, college or university.[30] These efforts often end up being traps because they're not totally under your control and if they see themself falling short in any of these areas, their self-worth plummets in a spiral of despair.[31]

The bodily changes associated with menopause, as we've mentioned, can badly affect those whose self-worth is pinned on how their body looks and what it can do. However, when you consider the neurological symptoms, you can also see how these might also affect other sources of self-worth for autistic people. For instance, some autistic people find that their job gives them a sense of identity, as well as a connection with other people who share that identity. They might find a sense of achievement and pride in excelling in their work.[32] The cognitive symptoms of menopause, like brain fog, might affect their ability to do their job, cutting off this source of self-worth and identity. This was very evident for some of our experts, as you'll see in Chapter 14 (page 145).

While non-autistic people might also experience threats to their self-worth during menopause (as you saw on page 40), autistic people are more likely to go into menopause with a lower, more fragile sense of self-worth, due to their experiences in the world. They may therefore have greater difficulties coping with the emotional impact of losing self-worth.

Autistic people are more likely to have struggled with periods and other reproductive transitions

We know that people who have struggled with difficult periods and previous reproductive transitions are more likely to experience difficulties at menopause.[33] This is worrisome for neurodivergent people as they seem to be unusually sensitive to monthly hormonal changes, and those that happen across the broader life course. One research team led by an autistic researcher talked to autistic people about their experiences of menstruating.[34] They found that autistic participants struggled with their emotions, executive function and sensory sensitivities to a greater extent during their period. Autistic people in that study also experienced more sensory overloads and meltdowns just before and during their periods, and were more likely to self-harm. Life became 'much more difficult to manage' during periods,[35] during which it became much 'harder to maintain control of the things that already take a lot of effort for us'.[36] A participant in another study said something similar about periods:

> " 'I feel everything that is happening, and I feel like it's just a lot of overwhelm. It might not be the worst pain ever, but I can't get my mind off of it. Just feeling every bit of bloating, feeling everything, my clothes don't fit right, and, you know, the skin changes, everything...'[37]

ADHDers also report profound impacts of monthly menstrual periods on their thought processes, emotions and ability to manage self-care.[38] It makes sense why monthly hormonal periods should affect neurodivergent people so much; it's those pesky hormonal fluctuations again, affecting the brain systems that underpin our senses, thoughts and emotions. This is also why other lifespan reproductive transitions, like pregnancy and the postnatal stage, can be so challenging. Here, again, autistic people report a heightening of their sensory sensitivities and emotions, and more frequent meltdowns and shutdowns.[39] As such, a history of difficult periods and other reproductive challenges might be cause for concern for autistic people and ADHDers when looking down the road ahead to menopause.

Throughout these experiences, unfortunately, many autistic people report feeling like their pain, discomfort and fear is dismissed or invalidated by healthcare professionals[40] (more on this in Chapter 20!). Similarly, previous healthcare encounters are also very important to wellbeing at menopause. If a person has received inadequate or even traumatizing healthcare during earlier reproductive stages, it stands to reason that they may not seek out support even if they're really struggling at menopause. This is even more concerning when we consider that autistic people might enter menopause with a greater burden of physical and mental illness.

Autistic people are more likely to enter menopause with poorer physical health

As a population, autistic people tend to have poorer physical health than non-autistic people. On average, autistic people in their 40s to 60s are more likely to have non-communicable diseases such as heart conditions (e.g. hypertension), respiratory conditions (e.g. asthma), gastrointestinal conditions (e.g. irritable bowel syndrome) and musculoskeletal conditions (e.g. arthritis).[41] Autistic people assigned female at birth are also more likely to have chronic illnesses that affect many organ systems, like fibromyalgia, Ehlers-Danlos syndrome and CFS/ME.[42] These are all conditions which stand to be affected by the changes of menopause, as discussed in Chapter 5 (pages 58–59), adding to the challenges autistic people may have to cope with during menopause.

Autistic people are more likely to enter menopause with poorer mental health

Autistic people are also more likely to be among those who enter menopause carrying a burden of current or historic mental illness.[43] Almost a third (32%) of autistic people assigned female at birth will be hospitalized for a severe mental illness before they reach the age of 25, in contrast to 5% of non-autistic counterparts.[44] Other statistics are equally startling: depression will be experienced by 37% of autistic people at some point in their lifespan, compared with 10.8% of non-autistic people.[45] Relatedly, one in three autistic people will experience suicidal thoughts in their lifetime,[46] in contrast to one in ten non-autistic people.[47]

At present, we do not know how many autistic people experience severe mental illness and suicidality at menopause, but as we mentioned in Chapter 5 (page 57), menopause is a time of vulnerability for the development of new mental illnesses and the worsening of pre-existing ones.[48] The role of sleep disturbance in poor mental health during menopause is notable,[49] given that sleep is often a problem for autistic people anyway and is already a factor in their mental illness.[50] These facts together suggest that autistic people may be a particularly vulnerable demographic for mental illness during menopause.

Factors associated with environment and life experiences

In the outer circle (Figure 7.1), we consider vulnerability factors to do with a person's environment and their life experiences.

Autistic people might have less access to information about menopause, and hence know less about it

As we discussed in Chapter 4 (pages 44–46), a person's psychological mindset in relation to menopause (their attitudes and feelings about it) is very important. We noted that greater resilience during menopause seems to be linked with having some sense of control over how you experience and manage your menopause symptoms and your health more broadly. A key aspect of feeling disempowered (less in control, not knowing what's going on) was having little knowledge about what to expect during menopause. While we noted that menopause education and awareness seems to be poor worldwide, studies indicate that many autistic people go into menopause with limited awareness of what to expect.[51] Some had a factual knowledge of symptoms like hot flushes, but were unprepared for how these would actually feel, and how profoundly symptoms would affect them. If we consider how people generally learn about menopause, one of the most common sources of information in non-autistic people is their friends.[52] Indeed, close friends are deemed by some women to be more reliable sources of information than online sources, and in some cases, more empathic than male partners.[53] Sadly, it's likely that many autistic people don't have access to this kind of supportive information-sharing about menopause since they are often ostracized by the people around them,[54] and this social isolation only tends to get worse with age.[55] The social stigma surrounding menopause means that these kinds of discussions might only take place in very intimate and trusting friendships, which, again, many autistic people do not have.

Another source of information about menopause is healthcare practitioners, but autistic people may be confounded by the barriers they face when seeking medical help.[56] There are a lot of hoops to jump through in order to speak to a doctor, from the phone call with a receptionist to secure an appointment, to enduring the sensory environment in the waiting room. When they finally reach that short appointment with the doctor, many autistic people find that they are misunderstood, disbelieved or dismissed; a traumatizing experience, especially when it happens many times over.[57] Autistic people who've had these kinds of experiences, including those who've previously had negative healthcare experiences in relation to gynaecological or reproductive health, might be understandably very reluctant to approach healthcare practitioners for information about menopause.

Autistic people might struggle to access support during menopause

Social support is important for coping with the trials and tribulations of life, for autistic and non-autistic people alike.[58] Menopause can definitely be one of those tribulations, and as we mentioned in Chapter 5 (page 55), some cisgender non-autistic women experience a kind of sisterhood, a camaraderie, with friends and acquaintances going through the same thing.[59] It seems very likely that autistic people might not be included in such circles of solidarity. As we've mentioned, autistic people often lack safe, trusting relationships with peers; indeed, sadly, friendships are sometimes a source of interpersonal victimization for them.[60] The experience of being autistic is, in the words of participants from a 2023 study, to be perpetually 'on the edge of it all'.[61]

Studies suggest that autistic women and AFAB (assigned female at birth) people can have an especially difficult time connecting with non-autistic women.[62] Cisgender female friendships have a tendency to be more socially complex than male friendships, based more around intimate conversations and emotional support (e.g. discussing challenges with romantic partners), while male friendships may be more structured around shared interests and activities (e.g. playing Dungeons and Dragons). Autistic women and AFAB people may be less likely to conform to gendered interests and expectations placed on them by society (e.g. to be a wife, mother), which can also create an 'invisible glass barrier'[63] between them and other women. This all means that when menopause arrives, they may not have friends they can talk to about it. While parents often play a crucial role as the friends and confidants of autistic adults,[64] chances are that by the time those autistic adults reach menopause, that vital support may no longer be available.

A seemingly obvious source of support at menopause is healthcare practitioners, who can offer a kind of tangible aid that friends and family cannot: access to treatment. However, this source of support requires autistic people to navigate a healthcare system which is inaccessible and which, as you'll hear from our experts in Chapter 20 (page 203), may have actually harmed them.[65] Although there are doubtless instances of good practice across the UK and the world, research suggests that in 2024, safe and supportive relationships between autistic people and their doctors are not the norm.[66]

Autistic people are more likely to have traumatic or stressful pasts

Unfortunately, autistic people are more likely to enter menopause with brains and bodies affected by the long-term consequences of stress and trauma. We are social animals, which is why the threat of negative social evaluation is a form of stress which affects people especially badly.[67] Sadly, negative perceptions of autism and autistic features mean that this threat is a persistent reality for autistic people, and it manifests in high rates of ostracism, exploitation, discrimination, persecution and victimization. Such victimization can be physical (e.g. being attacked), verbal (e.g. being verbally abused) or sexual (e.g. being assaulted or abused).[68]

Perhaps the most insidious forms of abuse are the kinds of emotional, physical and sexual abuse and exploitation which occur at the hands of people the person trusts, such as friends, romantic partners or family members.[69] We know that from childhood into adulthood, autistic people experience more of these kinds of incidents than non-autistic people. That's in addition to the more everyday stresses of sensory pain and fear,[70] being forced to fit into environments not suited for them.[71] We know that autistic people experience trauma from a wider range of experiences than those typically associated with post-traumatic stress disorder.[72] We also know that living as a marginalized group incurs its own impact on health. As we mentioned in Chapter 5 (pages 53–54), it's not just about the big things, but the slow drip of stigma, discrimination, inaccessible environments and unmet needs.[73] If you think back to how menopause 'unmasks' the effects of long-term trauma on the brain (page 53), then greater exposure to stress and trauma is likely a significant reason why autistic people might be intensely affected by the changes of menopause.

Autistic people are more likely to be affected by other inequalities
Autistic people are also vulnerable to another kind of adversity which affects brain and body: socioeconomic deprivation or poverty, which as we noted in Part 1 (pages 29, 42 and 53) is associated with earlier onset of menopause and more severe symptoms. Poverty is likely related to these aspects of menopause because people with less money have less access to information, support and resources to improve their health, and they tend to be more exposed to stress and trauma. Autistic people tend to leave school with lower qualifications, are less likely to take up or complete higher education, have less access to appropriate, sustainable employment, and are more at risk of homelessness.[74] While not all autistic people will be socioeconomically disadvantaged, for some it may be another factor tipping the scale against them and acting as a barrier to accessing information and care at menopause.

The cracks in the foundations
As you saw in the start of the chapter, these kinds of vulnerability factors are like cracks below the foundations of your Jenga tower. Some, like low self-worth, are relatively stable and not too problematic at

some points in your life, but might take on new significance during menopause. Most are related: for instance, it's likely that the poor mental and physical health of autistic people is partly stress-related. There are a few additional factors which might make menopause especially challenging for some autistic people, such as other forms of neurodivergence or marginalized identities, and we'll come back to these in later chapters.

This may have been a difficult read. It seems extremely cruel that many of these difficult life circumstances – physical and mental illness, trauma – continue to play out their effects across the lifespan. We believe it's important to know why menopause might be harder for autistic people, as for other marginalized or disadvantaged groups. If you are autistic, we hope that it helps you to understand that there are very legitimate reasons why you might be struggling more than others during the menopausal transition, and it's not your fault – moreover, it doesn't mean you can't be helped. Similarly, if you're someone who supports autistic people, professionally or otherwise, it may help to understand the very real differences in the mind, brain and body which could make menopause more challenging and which need to be accommodated in supports.

Chapter 8

The bigger picture

Autistic people navigating midlife

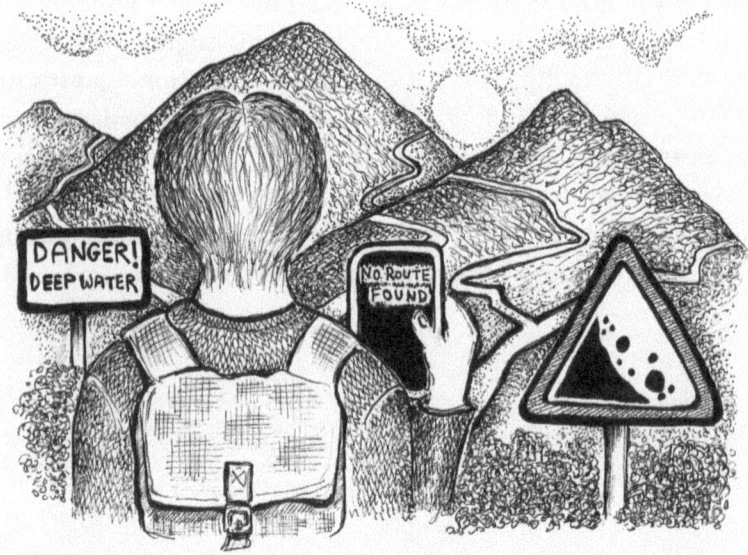

Midlife can be a bit of a bumpy ride. In Chapter 4 (pages 47–48), we talked about the many changes and pressures that midlife brings, changes which affect people's relationships, and their lives at home and at work. The metaphor of the sandwich generation illustrates how you might find yourself in the middle with responsibility for and demands from both younger and older generations,[1] from family and at work. There may also be relationship stress with your partner or spouse, ongoing health issues, and perhaps worries about the future. Then menopause comes along on top of this multi-layered midlife sandwich.

It's hard enough for anyone but what of those who struggle with change? We didn't specifically ask our autistic experts about the other events happening in their lives around menopause, but the pressures they were experiencing at midlife kept creeping into the conversation. Here Tara very clearly shows her experience of being in between two generations:

> " 'I just could not work out how to accommodate all the conflicting needs... elderly parents, teenage sons, conflicting needs, overwhelming demands, lack of SEN [special educational needs] support, fighting the SEN system... I think that would be overwhelming [even] if you didn't have your own issues on top of it!' TARA

Tara's quote also indicates that there might be additional midlife challenges that autistic people are more likely to experience, as we'll go on to explore.

The generation below: challenges around children

Not all of our autistic experts had children, but several did. Neurodivergent people are more likely to have children who are also neurodivergent, as was the case for some of our experts. Bridie, navigating the emotional turmoil of her own perimenopause as an undiagnosed autistic person, was fighting for her two teenage children to be diagnosed as autistic, 'getting thrown from one paediatrician to the next'. The Cat, too, was supporting an autistic son through secondary school, 'putting him first' while 'this stuff was going on with me in the background'. Many parents, like Bridie and The Cat, advocate fiercely for years to access support for their children.[2] Although some autistic parents will encounter menopause when their children are still young, most menopausal people with children will be parenting teenagers or young adults. This creates a whole set of further challenges, as Sally described:

> " 'My children were in the throes of their teenage years and they were... while I can theorize that it's very healthy for them to break away from their parents... it just felt like a massive rejection at the time.'

The turbulence of life with teenagers has been a consistent thread in the conversations we've had with autistic people over the years. From the 'raging arguments', to being unable to 'be the way [my autistic son] needs me to be because of my own challenges',[3] some of these autistic parents reported that after having taken care of everyone else, they had 'no energy left for me'.[4]

As hard as having children at home can be, some parents mourn and dread the day they leave home. One of our research participants said:

> 'You've spent your whole life raising them up to the point where they are decent company and then they leave... it can make you feel like you have no purpose, nothing left in life.'[5]

But not all autistic people are parents at midlife. Some are childfree by choice,[6] while others might have liked to have had children but never had the opportunity. Both of these states can be emotionally challenging in different ways. Not having a child, particularly as a woman, is another way in which a person can be othered from their peers, pitied and/or judged.[7] Furthermore, for some non-autistic individuals, the signalled loss of reproductive opportunity with menopause can bring complex emotions, including grief and regret. Lachman and her colleagues, who talked about the crossroads of midlife (pages 47–48), suggest that people without children may have lower life satisfaction, overall, in these midlife years.

Because older autistic people are virtually absent from research, we know very little about how older autistic people without children feel about not being parents. Some autistic people we've interviewed, however, have expressed some of these challenging feelings, where menopause evokes a 'deep mourning'[8] for lost opportunities and lives they could have had, sentiments which have been echoed in other published work with autistic people at menopause.[9] One autistic woman said that she keenly felt the weight of societal expectations that she'd never fulfilled, and it set her apart from other people:

> 'I think society places a lot of, you know, how you're supposed to be... you're supposed to do this in this part of your life, you know, get your education, your career, relationships, marriage and children and things

like that... it can be hard being with other people because I feel like they won't understand where I'm coming from... It's a bit harder to relate to people of my age, because they have children [or even] grandchildren ... I guess I'm a bit conscious of [the things I haven't done]. I already find it difficult to talk and communicate and I suppose that is an added kind of thing, you know?'[10]

The generation above: parenting your parent

As we noted in Chapter 4 (page 48), for many people midlife brings a particular reversal in our relationship with our parents. The support that has typically flowed from parent to child gradually reverses as our parents age and encounter illness and infirmity, and eventually, we lose them. In the midst of struggling with menopause and major life changes of their own, Spike encountered increasing tension with their brother:

> 'Mum was diagnosed with dementia around the time that I started menopause... we had to sell her house to pay for nursing care, and there was a lot of stuff that we had to pull together to do. He wanted me to step up more. He doesn't get it... it made me feel really guilty about the fact that I couldn't "step up" more.'

Other autistic people we've talked to described the difficulties of taking care of parents through the illnesses of old age; some felt guilty for struggling, and even more so if they lost their temper when under extreme strain.[11] Others went through menopause and midlife in amongst a sea of grief for a parent – a grief which could be additionally confusing if alexithymia was in the mix. One autistic woman said:

> 'I struggled really badly to understand what emotion I was feeling at times, and like, I was feeling grief but I felt it as anger, or just not as things that I expected it to be, and I couldn't explain to my husband what I was feeling or why I was angry or why I was crying suddenly, and I didn't understand.'[12]

It's important to recognize that for some autistic people, the loss of parental support is particularly significant. For many, parents are their confidants, their (only) friends and companions, and their sources of emotional and practical support.[13] We don't know exactly how many autistic people live with their parents in their 30s, 40s and 50s, but we know that 76% of autistic people between the ages of 16 and 64 years live with their parents. That's a rate higher than seen in people with physical disabilities, learning disabilities or mental illnesses.[14] The loss of their parents puts these individuals at risk of living on the street, couch-surfing or living in temporary or unsafe housing.[15] It may also drastically affect their ability to manage self-care, to hold a job and to cope with everyday life.

Crucially, we must however remember that not all autistic people enjoy supportive relationships with their parents. This was the case for a number of our autistic experts. For some of them, midlife entailed or continued a painful process of coping and healing from painful and/or traumatic parental relationships. Bereavement of an estranged parent can activate old wounds, spark complex emotions including guilt, regret and anger, and can be especially difficult when other people do not recognise the significance of the loss. This kind of bereavement might, as such, feel equally devastating and bewildering as that of a loving parent, as another change to navigate during midlife.

Slammed from the side: work-related challenges

Sadly, autistic people across the world appear to face similar kinds of barriers to employment.[16] Autistic people who are unable to work, for whatever reason, can really struggle.[17] Though they might not experience changes in this part of their lives at midlife, they might feel something of the sense of difference described by our autistic participant above, who struggled to relate to people with children and careers.

Not all of our autistic experts were working at midlife, but several who were described changes in their working lives. Some, like Katie and Tara, had to leave their jobs because they were struggling with mental health and/or burnout. Others, like Anne, were made redundant, and had to find work at reduced hours to fit her needs. Some, like Alice and Spike, moved from traditional forms of employment into self-employment or freelance work. Daisy, too, described needing to 'scale back'; having previously been able to stand up to senior management, she found herself 'not able to take on that kind of level of people any more'.

These kinds of experience aren't all that uncommon. We know that a lot of people leave the workforce in midlife, with menopausal symptoms and other midlife demands, such as caring for ageing parents, contributing to this withdrawal.[18] While some manage to remain at work, they might find themselves burning out through their efforts to compensate for perceived shortcomings, or struggling with the stigma or discrimination attached to ageing, especially as a woman or someone assigned female at birth. Autistic participants in our previous studies had a lot to say about this. One woman pointed out how the different marginalized aspects of her identity might be interacting in the way her workplace treated her:

66 'I had a high impact, high value job and am now treated like dirt. I am left puzzling whether this is because I am a woman, an ageing woman, or an ageing autistic woman who has been treated for cancer... I now feel completely overwhelmed and undervalued.'[19]

Importantly, not all work-related changes at midlife are negative; several of our autistic experts said that the changes they'd made at midlife had improved their quality of life, and some had pursued exciting new pathways. One autistic lady we spoke to said that following the turbulence of menopause, she was 'really hitting my stride... [by my] early to late 50s, I was doing better than I ever had in my life!'[20] It's important to hear about these kinds of positive experiences which might be less talked about, and we'll come back to them later in this book (Chapters 18 and 19).

It's worth thinking again about those autistic people who do leave the workforce, though, as some will during menopause. Autistic people who retire can struggle with the loss of routine, structure and social connection.[21] Another thing that people can lose, with retirement, changes at work and other midlife changes, is a sense of identity, purpose and self-worth. This is vital for wellbeing, and several of our autistic experts expressed that their challenges at work had shaken this source of self-worth and purpose. Claire, who eventually needed to withdraw from a social work career she'd begun during midlife, was distressed when she told us:

❝ 'I no longer feel capable of being a social worker... I feel lost and upset... I like being a social worker. I'm good at being a social worker. It's who I am. It's what I do... people talk about having a midlife crisis. I have an identity crisis. I've lost my identity. I don't know who I am any more. I don't know who I want to be.'

Shaking foundations: relationship changes at midlife

Naturally, the kinds of external stressors and psychological changes that people experience at midlife can put immense strain on relationships with partners and spouses, who will often be navigating their own midlife changes. Relationship breakdown is common enough in this period that it's been dubbed 'grey divorce'.[22] Of course, not all autistic people will be in a romantic relationship at midlife but some of our autistic experts enjoyed supportive relationships which had weathered and matured over time, and continued to do so. In Tara's words, 'we've been together for over 20 years, so we've renegotiated and moved around each other and grown and all this sort of stuff'.

For some non-autistic people, the changes in sex drive (libido) which often accompany menopause are a significant challenge for relationships.[23] Most people find their sex drive changes across their lifespan, and so some of our experts found it 'very lucky' that as their own libido decreased, so did that of their partner. This was not the case for all of our experts, who found their libido increasingly out of sync with that of their partner. In these instances, lowered libido and other physical symptoms of menopause had severe negative impacts on relationships. The negative impact of menopause and midlife stress on intimate relationships has been something mentioned many times by autistic people who've spoken to us. More broadly, the impact of menopausal symptoms on relationships with close others is something we'll come back to again throughout the chapters in Part 3.

Autistic people have also told us about other major relationship changes at midlife, such as Suzi, who escaped domestic abuse, and participants from our previous studies, who talked about divorce and relationship breakdowns at midlife. Conversely, some autistic people have mentioned new obsessions related to other people and relationships. Alice mentioned developing 'the most enormous, all-consuming crush' on a colleague, the kind of obsession she'd experienced in her youth, which had come back in full force during menopause. For Alice, this 'wasn't fun... it was very intrusive... I felt like a teenager and it was just crazy'. Alice got through it with her marriage intact. In contrast, in our research, one participant told us that they blamed 'menopausal madness'[24] for an impulsive and ill-judged marriage, as they explained:

> 'I look back at it now and there were like major red flags in this situation and I... chose to... Either not read them or not regard them, I can't recall just now what was going on there... But I didn't pay attention in a way that I should have. Maybe I just wanted something really exciting to happen in my life and that I was running out of time for it, I don't know.'[25]

The weight of health and the future

As we mentioned earlier (pages 52–9), menopause and other age-related changes, as well as the impacts of long-term stress, mean that some people will have to cope with health conditions at midlife. Almost all of our autistic experts mentioned health complaints which started or were aggravated at this time. Some, like Daisy, Sally and Anne, had chronic health conditions (e.g. fibromyalgia, chronic fatigue and hypermobility) which worsened during midlife. Daisy was very unlucky: in addition to her fatigue, she had to fight breast cancer, and developed 'overwhelming allergies' and a rare immune system condition. She noted how expensive it had been to manage her health, since the UK health system 'doesn't work for people with systemic conditions that go across all of your body'. Sadly, this is something we've heard from many people with complex health conditions.[26] Managing your own health takes a lot of work, cognitively and emotionally, as well as financially.

When they see the signs of ageing in themselves and their loved ones, midlife is a time where many people start to think about their later years. The future and old age are things that many people fear, but they are likely to be particularly frightening for autistic people.[27] Some fear the thought of having to live in environments which won't accommodate their sensory needs and routines, and some, as we've mentioned, fear the loss of the people who love and support them.

Going through health problems yourself, or supporting a partner through theirs, can shake up these kinds of fears, as one autistic woman told us:

66 'I suddenly realized, oh shit, my husband could die, in fact my husband IS going to die before me probably, and I'm going to be on my own.'[28]

We've had autistic people tell us that the experience of menopause during midlife is like a 'perfect storm',[29] a time where issues and demands seem to pile on all at once. Even without menopause in the mix, midlife can be a formidable time. The potential scale of unmet needs is all the more worrying when we consider the tiny fraction of funding spent on services and supports for older autistic adults.

Chapter 9

The importance of knowing

When menopause comes before an autism diagnosis

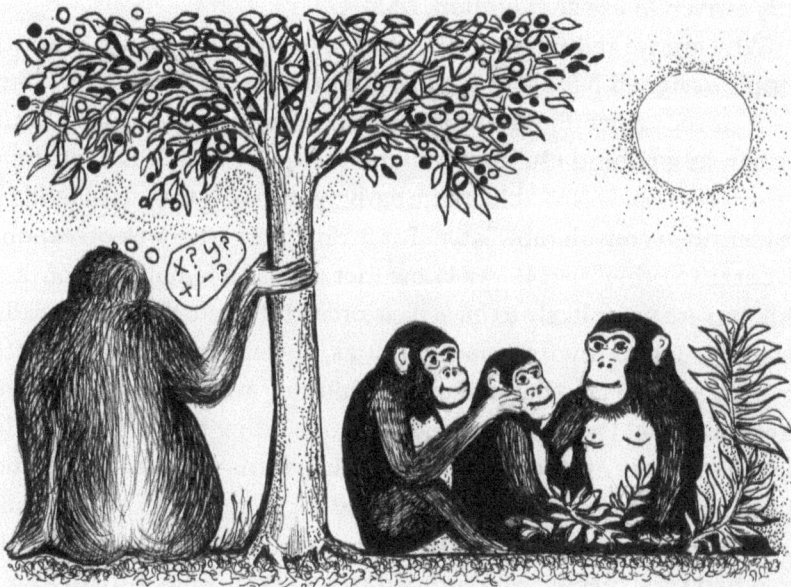

The concept of autism hasn't been around long in the scheme of things.[1] You might know something about how it came about: a couple of blokes in the 1940s, jotting down notes about the little boys they were observing, either side of the Second World War. The history of autism is murky in parts and beyond the scope of this book, but as an official diagnosis, 'infantile autism' arrived in the *Diagnostic and Statistical Manual of Mental Disorders* (DSM: the handbook used by many psychiatrists) in 1980.[2]

'Infantile autism' looked very different to what we think of as autism today. Children had to show 'pervasive lack of responsiveness to other people', 'gross deficits in language development' and 'bizarre responses to various aspects of the environment'.[3] Ironically, given the inflexibility that people often ascribe to autism, there was no allowance for deviation from the precise diagnostic criteria; each and every one had to be met, and these differences had to be present before 30 months of age. The concept of autism as a spectrum only arrived in the 1990s, at which point individuals could be diagnosed with Asperger syndrome or the rather unpleasant-sounding catch-all for unusual cases, 'pervasive developmental disorder not otherwise specified'.[4] The fact that autistic people may learn to mask their autism, such that it might not be observable to the casual observer, only arrived in the 2013 edition, DSM-5.[5]

Why are we telling you this? Well, essentially because autistic people assigned female at birth, born prior to the year 2000, often went unrecognized and undiagnosed. What we now know about autism in girls and children assigned female at birth is that their autism is often less visible in the early years, such that they tend to be identified considerably later.[6] Far from a 'pervasive lack of responsiveness to other people', we know that girls and female-presenting children are more likely to have passionate interests that are socially related, such as environmental issues, social justice, or interests focused around another person. As children, autistic girls are more likely to exist at the fringes of social groups rather than being overtly excluded. Some are exceptionally proficient maskers, adopting the speech mannerisms, body language and social customs of other children. At that time, adults around those undiagnosed autistic children had very specific, stereotyped views about what autism looks like, informed by films such as 1988's *Rain Man*. Autistic children with learning disabilities would typically be picked up, but many individuals with good language and average to high IQs simply didn't fit that picture. The adults who would normally raise queries about a child (e.g. their parents, teachers, even doctors) might have just labelled them as a bit 'quirky'.

As a result, for decades, autistic girls and female-presenting children with average to high IQs were missing from research, and from clinical descriptions. Even from the 1990s onwards, when we were starting to understand autism much better, we were still catching up from the many years where girls, women and people assigned female at birth were simply absent from the literature which informs diagnosis and support for autistic people.

To give you a scale of how many people grew up undiagnosed in those years, you might think about a statistic that's often touted around: that 1% of the UK's population are known to be autistic (1 in 100 people). A recent study suggests a further 1–2% of the UK population, predominantly older people assigned female at birth, are undiagnosed autistic.[7] We often call these individuals the 'lost generation'[8] and those born pre-1990s are now growing into midlife and older age.

What's it like to grow up undiagnosed?

Since more and more people are learning they're autistic in adulthood, we're coming to know a bit more about their lives and experiences. In all our years working with autistic people, one incredible analogy has stuck in our minds, beautifully reflecting the realities of growing up undiagnosed and of masking. A participant in our menopause research was telling us about this invisible aura of difference which surrounded them as a child and made other kids keep their distance. Using the analogy of a zoo, they said:

> 'In the primate enclosures live the bonobos, and those are the neurotypicals. They are a very social group, they do a lot of grooming, have very strong social hierarchies... they do all their bonobo things in their bonobo kind of way.
>
> And in that same enclosure are two or three orangutans... the neurodivergent people. They're also primates so on certain levels they get what the bonobos are doing, but orangutans are solitary, they don't do bonobo group things, it's just completely foreign to their mentality.
>
> My whole life, I've been an orangutan among the bonobos. I observe the bonobos and I notice under x circumstances they do y thing, so I mask by doing y thing when I think x circumstances are going on. But, since they are bonobos, they know this is an *X-SQUARED* circumstance and they should do *y-1 thing*, and I don't know that and so my mask is always a bit crooked.
>
> It's always felt like that; it's like I watch, I watch, I watch, but I'm always

still an orangutan, you know, I can't quite... get there. And they know it, they know it. They look at me and they think "wow, that's not a bonobo"... if neurotypicals have an instinct to their bones, it's the "them and us" one. They know who's them and who's us.'[9]

There are now many, many studies which confirm just the same kinds of experience.[10] Growing up as just a bit 'odd', the lost generation would have received little, if any, support or understanding from others. They typically speak of struggling academically at mainstream school, of vicious and chronic bullying, and the challenges of finding and coping with work. They speak of the strain and stress of being that solitary orangutan trying to speak bonobo: of their conscious and unconscious masking, their challenges managing platonic and non-platonic relationships, with some falling prey to exploitation and abuse, and others baffled by the gulf of difference separating them from others. They are often people with complex mental health histories, individuals whose anxiety and depression were resistant to any (un-adapted) treatments thrown at them.

Many of our autistic experts described experiences like these. Florence, for instance, said their teenage years were 'traumatic':

" 'I didn't know why I didn't have many friends. I was diagnosed with anxiety and depression. I was put on Valium when I was 14, but that made me feel worse. I thought I must be a horrible person to not have friends. I thought I must be a weak person because I found some things hard.'

Florence's thoughts and feelings are echoed consistently by hundreds of late-diagnosed autistic participants across many studies. Their self-narratives are ones of 'failure', of being 'defective', 'broken', 'weird', 'stupid', 'shit at life' or 'lacking as a person'.[11] They also often blame themselves for being bullied or abused by others. It's not surprising that late-diagnosed autistic people have higher suicide rates and poorer mental health.[12]

Menopause unmasking neurodivergence

If you think back to previous chapters, you'll remember that mental illness, lifetime adversity and socioeconomic disadvantage are associated with more severe menopause symptoms. The cards are indeed stacked against undiagnosed autistic people when they experience a menopause which doesn't look and feel like that of neurotypical descriptions; not knowing about their autism, they may have no explanation for why their menopause might differ. In fact, there seems to be a two-way relationship between neurodivergence and menopause (Figure 9.1):

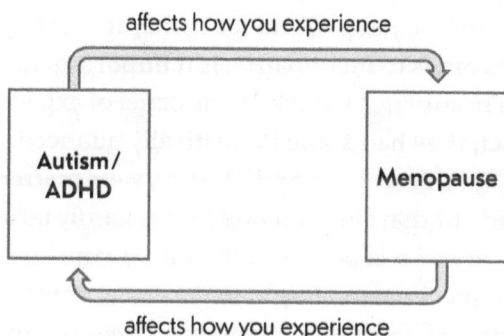

affects how you experience

Autism/ADHD — Menopause

affects how you experience

Figure 9.1 *Reciprocal relationships between neurodivergence and menopause*

Autistic people we've spoken to have said that their previous coping strategies and masks stopped working at menopause.[13] Aspects of autism and ADHD, such as difficulties with executive function, became magnified; sensory sensitivities increased or emerged from nowhere; and emotions became more intense. We'll talk about all these aspects in detail in Part 3, but changes in the way people experience their neurodivergence meant that suddenly, in the words of one participant:

> 'It was like visible autism to the max... it was like autism going... with too many toppings' (laughing).[14]

In this way, some people said that menopause led them to their autism diagnosis 'because I've stopped being able to cope with my life, the life I was able to cope with before'.[15]

Why is it important to know you're autistic before entering menopause?

Realizing a late-life autistic identity is an emotional thing, and it's not uncommon for people to experience grief and anger, thinking of the missed chances and suffering that might have been averted.[16] That said, for many people, it's not an exaggeration to say that knowing about their autism is 'the single most important thing that has happened in [their] life'.[17] Late-diagnosed autistic people appear to agree when they say that understanding this crucial fact about themselves allows them to be more self-compassionate, to better self-advocate and protect themselves, to explain themselves to others, find their tribe in other autistic people, and for some, access formal support.

So, when it comes to menopause, is it important to know beforehand that you're autistic? We asked our panel of experts and as we'd come to expect, they had some fantastically nuanced answers.

Some, like Tara, Bassai Sho and The Cat, were matter-of-fact. Bassai Sho pointed out that since menopause is hardly talked about and she only knew her own experience, she wasn't sure how it differed to what a neurotypical person might experience, or whether it would have been different had she known about her autism beforehand. Tara, postmenopause, said that since there had been so little information about autistic menopause at the time she went through it, she wasn't sure how much knowing about her autism would have helped her, though she hoped 'the next generation of women coming to this book that'll have these different voices, and different stories... can start making sense of and understanding their own experience' (we hope so, too!). The Cat reflected that while knowing about her autism didn't make much difference to her at menopause, it might be important for some:

66 'I could see somebody be in a position where they'd lose close relationships through their own behaviour and not understanding why they're doing it. I could see it ruining lives. I could think you could end up living under a bridge, to be honest.' THE CAT

This is the kind of sentiment expressed by our other autistic experts. Anne and Sally, who'd gone through menopause undiagnosed, said:

" 'I don't think I've ever felt so confused and out of control.' ANNE

" 'I honestly thought I was going mad sometimes. I was very upset a lot of the time because I didn't know what was wrong with me.' SALLY

Ann and Lily, likewise, expressed how 'scary' and 'baffling' it could be to go through menopause undiagnosed, both pointing out how difficult that would make it to seek appropriate help and find people who understood:

" 'I knew nothing about, you know, the normal kind of sensory things that autistic people experience anyway, and then to have those amplified [at menopause]... I wouldn't have sailed through it, but I could have dealt with it better [if I'd known]. And just even knowing what else was going on and being able to say to somebody, this is what's going on, or go look for help or support or anything like that, you know. But when you, when you can't articulate what's going on for yourself, it's really difficult.' LILY

" 'It's like being an alien on earth and you don't know why you're an alien and everyone else isn't an alien. So imagine that, and then going through menopause, it'd be a really difficult time. I think it'd be really important that people know first, because I think it would help them through navigating their menopause journey, getting the right help or support or input or, you know, being able to research a bit... or find other autistic people who are also going through it because, you know, you're going to feel more akin to that, aren't you.' ANN

Several of our experts felt that knowing about their autism would have allowed them to be more self-compassionate at menopause and other times in their lives:

" 'I wouldn't have felt that I was even madder than I thought I was... it's really important that young people get diagnosed as soon as they possibly can... My children... say, "this makes so much sense, Mum. Everything makes so much more sense. I know I'm not just mad." You know, they smile that they've got a diagnosis, rather than being depressed.' BRIDIE

" 'I probably would have been a lot kinder on myself, more understanding of why everything seemed magnified, everything seemed... you know, when I speak to other people, menopause would be an annoyance, but not quite the same [scale]. And I think maybe, maybe I wouldn't have felt like, I mean, I really felt like I was going mad. I think some of that was just because, for the whole of my life I felt like something wasn't quite right [with me] anyway. So [at menopause] it was just like an added concrete block of weirdness on top of everything else.' JANET

Some added that knowing might have helped them draw on coping skills or find new strategies, as well as reassurance that this time would end:

" 'It [menopause] would be easier because then you'd be kinder to your-self a lot quicker. And you, you would understand that this was okay, this is pretty horrible, but actually, it was a phase of life and this was why it was happening and this was why it was you were experiencing it as you were.' KATIE

" 'There are things that I do and things that I find difficult. Knowing that I'm autistic makes it easier for me to cope in the sense that I don't just think I'm a terrible, useless person. And also easier for me to find coping strategies because I can think, "Oh, okay, well, I know that I'm autistic and I know that I have coping strategies for these things. And yes, menopause is making them worse. But because I know I'm autistic, I know I have some idea of how to deal with these things." So I think it's just generally true that knowing that I'm autistic makes it easier for me to deal with things like emotional dysregulation.' ALICE

Some of our experts, like Suzi, pointed out that knowing about their autism would have helped them advocate for themselves in health-care. Daisy, too, suggested that knowing about her autism would have helped in relationships generally, and that knowing about menopause broadly, as well as menopause as an autistic person, could have prepared her for the worsening of her health:

" 'For me, knowing about it in my life generally explains so much. Not having to apologize for being me and not having to apologize for being quite straight speaking, and just say, "you know, I am straight speaking, don't take offence," rather than having to just apologize all the time... I think with the menopause, I think it would have been very useful. You know, it would be very useful to know about the menopause [laughing] and then it would be very useful to know about autism, because I didn't know about either really. And the combination of the two and the fact that it would tip me over the edge, having the combination of the two with all my immune system stuff as well, that would have been very useful.'

Although late-diagnosed autistic people tend to have poorer mental health,[18] there isn't a straightforward correlation between age at diagnosis and quality of life in adulthood. It seems likely that the benefits conferred by knowing you are autistic actually come from other factors, like growing up with a positive sense of autistic identity and access to a wider autistic community,[19] which are more likely for young people diagnosed today. Nevertheless, autistic people across studies, and those we've spoken to, are resolute that knowing about their autism has improved their quality of life. On the whole, we conclude that early diagnosis is absolutely imperative to increase the likelihood of positive health and wellbeing outcomes for autistic people and that knowing about your autism before menopause is important for forward planning, self-compassion, coping and accessing support, all highlighted by our experts as essential aspects of coping (Chapter 17).

Chapter 10

Menopause and other forms of neurodivergence

Learning disabilities, ADHD and AuDHD

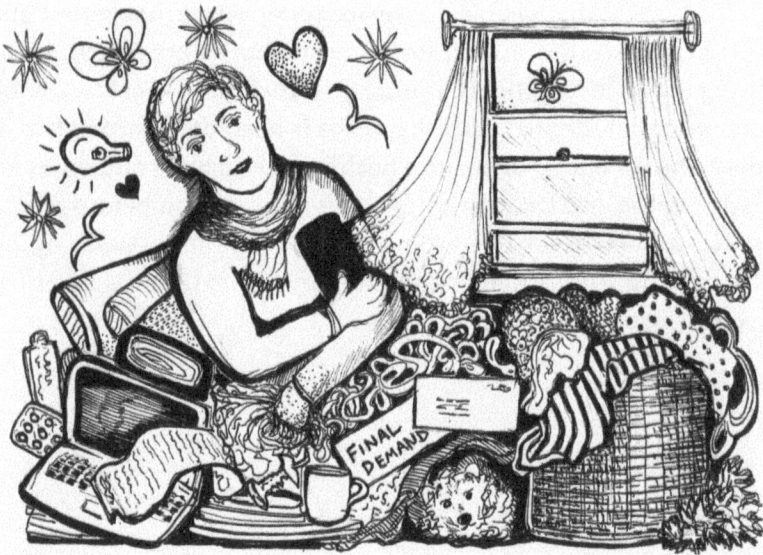

There are many ways of being neurodivergent. Some forms of neurodivergence are somewhat 'encapsulated'. For instance, specific learning difficulties like dyslexia, dyspraxia and dyscalculia are believed to primarily involve certain cognitive domains (e.g. reading, coordination, maths) without affecting the person's IQ or broader aspects of their functioning. Others, like autism, ADHD and learning disabilities, colour the person's experience and interactions with the world more globally. Neurodevelopmental differences are sociable and generous fellows – you rarely get one without (at least) one extra coming along for the ride!

What they all share, though, is that they are neurological differences and could be affected by the neurological ripples caused by menopause. In this chapter we'll consider, in a menopause context, two forms of neurodivergence which commonly co-occur with autism. Learning disability is an area where we know relatively little in a menopause context, while we'll spend more time in the growing research field that is ADHD and menopause.

Learning disabilities

A learning disability (LD; also known as intellectual disability in the USA) means having 'reduced intellectual ability' (essentially like IQ: struggling with complex or abstract reasoning, understanding new or complex information), coupled with 'reduced ability to cope independently'.[1] It differs from specific learning difficulties that affect particular types of learning, like dyslexia, but which do not affect someone's overall intellectual ability.

We're not sure how many autistic people have a LD but estimations range from 30% to around 50%. However, there are different degrees of LD.[2] A person with a 'mild' LD might be pretty independent but still need help in some areas of their lives, like planning a journey or filling in forms. A person with a 'severe' or 'profound' LD might have 'high support needs' as part of their autism diagnosis: they might need more extensive help with staying safe, feeding, personal care and hygiene, and may have great difficulties expressing themselves and understanding others.

Autistic people with LD, especially those whose LD are classified as 'severe' or 'profound', are often not included in research because it can be difficult to ensure that they fully understand and consent to participate. This means they get even less of a voice in issues concerning autistic people. Our studies so far were unfortunately inaccessible for these individuals. However, autistic people we spoke to continuously reflected on how difficult menopause might be for people with even greater difficulties understanding available information about menopause, and who might have greater difficulty expressing their pain and distress.[3] We know that this is true of monthly periods, through reports from those who support autistic people with 'severe' or 'profound' LD.[4] While not necessarily understanding what is happening to them, autistic people with LD seem to experience the heightening of existing challenges with emotion, thinking and sensory sensitivities reported by other autistic people,[5] but are dependent on others recognizing and correctly interpreting their signs of distress and pain, and knowing how to help.

There are ways that people with different degrees of LD can be enabled to participate in research if they want to,[6] but no research has yet managed to explore the menopausal experiences of these autistic individuals. Research in non-autistic people with 'mild' to 'moderate' LD suggests that they, too, can struggle with feeling uninformed and confused about menopause.[7] It can be very hard, if you do not fully understand what's happening, to tolerate the fluctuating nature of symptoms. Participants who spoke to Langer-Shapland and colleagues experienced a lot of worry about heavy, irregular periods, asking, 'Will it happen today? Is it going to come back?'[8] They found it helpful when provided with accessible information about menopause but still struggled to fully understand it. Like autistic people we've spoken to, non-autistic people with LD felt that conversation and social support around menopause was important in helping them cope. We agree with their emphasizing that:

> 'It should be more outspoken and not hushed away, not like put in a dark box.'[9]

While Langer-Shapland's work with non-autistic people with LD shows very important steps forwards, they focused on traditional menopause symptoms, like hot flushes. We don't know at present whether people with LD might experience a heightening of existing difficulties with thought processes, emotions and sensory sensitivities – and whether these might be a problem for autistic people with LD at menopause. We do know that over-prescribing medication can be a serious problem for autistic people with LD, who are often unable to advocate for themselves. Researchers point out that this could easily be a threat to their wellbeing at menopause, if doctors do not understand the nature of their difficulties.[10] Autistic people with LD and complex needs are often infantilized when it comes to sexual and reproductive health,[11] so we need to know more about how to support and empower them through later life transitions.

Attention-deficit/hyperactivity disorder (ADHD)

ADHD is diagnosed on the basis of two features: inattention and hyperactivity/impulsivity. People can be diagnosed with the predominantly inattentive subtype, the hyperactive subtype, or the combined subtype. The inattentive subtype used to be called attention deficit disorder (ADD), so where we talk about ADHD, this term includes inattentive-subtype people who might have previously received a diagnosis of ADD.

Actually, the name is a bit of a misnomer since ADHDers do not have a deficit or deficiency of attention. Rather, they struggle to control their attention. The 'inattentive' features of ADHD mean having a brain that is forgetful and constantly distracted by a 'constant barrage of thoughts and sensations'[12] around you, so you struggle to focus on a conversation or task, even when you really want to and know you have to. On the flip side, ADHDers also have times of hyper-focus, times of attention in abundance, a state of 'flow' where they can be immensely productive but lost to time, the world around them and their bodily needs.[13] Frustratingly, it's impossible to summon hyper-focus at will, or switch it on and off. One community advocate explained it as follows:

> 'Everyone with ADHD knows that they can "get in the zone" at least four or five times a day. When they are in the zone, they have no impairments, and the executive function deficits they may have had before entering the zone disappear. People with ADHD know that they are bright and clever, but they are never sure whether their abilities will show up when they need them. The fact that symptoms and impairments come and go throughout the day is the defining trait of ADHD. It makes the condition mystifying and frustrating.'[14]

The hyperactive/impulsive features of ADHD are much more noticeable to outside observers, and tend to be more common in people assigned male at birth (this is one reason males are diagnosed earlier).[15] ADHDers describe having 'exceptional reserves of energy', 'a brain with a thousand tentacles going at once'.[16] While some say this brings fun experiences and helps their productivity,[17] hyperactive/impulsive tendencies can also bring about unintended consequences, resulting in ADHDers being physically hurt, traumatized, socially ostracized or in trouble with the law. It can be physically painful or nauseating for ADHDers to not act on the impulses and thoughts which cross their brains, and they often concentrate better when they're moving or fidgeting, as one research participant commented:

> 66 'I call it "giving my monkey something to juggle"... all the stimulation is actually helping me feel very calm. The monkey is very busy at this time so there's no interference.'[18]

ADHD desperately needs a rebrand. Just like autism, it has traditionally been understood through a biomedical, pathologizing lens, without recognizing the wonderful qualities of ADHDers: their sense of wonder, curiosity and fascination, their empathy, energy and creativity.[19] One ADHD community theorist describes the ADHD brain as 'a unique and special creation that regulates attention and emotions in different ways... a nervous system that works well using its own set of rules'.[20] It follows naturally, of course, that much like autistic people, ADHDers will struggle in an unaccommodating world.

Shared features and experiences with autistic people

We like to think of ADHDers as 'neurological cousins' (p.7) to autistic people, a phrase from a paper pointing out the shared genetic factors and overlapping cognitive and emotional similarities between autism and ADHD.[21] Autistic people and ADHDers have so much in common. For instance, ADHDers also experience sensory differences, including over- and under-sensitivity to sounds, smells, light and colours, tastes, textures and touches. Like many autistic people, ADHDers experience their emotions as intense, overwhelming and fast-changing, and can experience hyper-empathy for others.[22] At the same time, many struggle with alexithymia and interoceptive awareness of their bodily signals.[23]

Although not unique to ADHD, you may hear ADHDers talk of

rejection sensitivity dysphoria (RSD): feelings of devastation, despair and self-loathing which they experience when anticipating or experiencing social rejection.[24] Importantly, RSD isn't a phenomenon that ADHDers experience 'all in their heads'; sadly, it's a reality. Public perceptions of ADHD range from scepticism (the 'ADHD is a fashionable excuse for laziness and bad behaviour' crowd), to stereotyping ADHDers as 'disruptive', 'unreliable' or 'deviants'.[25] Like autistic people, ADHDers are very often socially ostracized, discriminated against, exploited or abused. Unsurprisingly, they also have very high rates of masking, chronic physical illness, mental illness, burnout and suicide.

If we think about ADHD in a menopause context, you can see that ADHDers are likely to arrive at menopause with many of the same disadvantages: pre-existing neurological differences in attention, executive function and emotion; difficulties with emotions and interoceptive awareness; bodies aged by lifetime trauma; and mental and physical illnesses that might be worsened by menopause. Just like autistic people, historic under-recognition of ADHD in people assigned female at birth[26] means that many will enter menopause not knowing they are neurodivergent, instead seeing themselves as 'stupid', 'lazy' or 'broken'.[27]

'I dropped all the plates I'd been struggling to keep spinning'

There's virtually no published research on ADHDers' experiences of menopause, though reviews on reproductive hormones and ADHD highlight that the menopausal transition could, theoretically, heighten difficulties with cognition and emotion.[28] However, ADDitude magazine surveyed the menopause experiences of their readership, around 1500 people who'd been formally diagnosed or self-identified with ADHD.[29] Ninety-four per cent of participants said that challenges associated with ADHD had worsened during the menopausal transition, and strikingly, around half said that ADHD affected them more during menopause than it ever had in their lives to date.

Interestingly, like some of our autistic experts in Chapter 1, ADHDers in the ADDitude survey were most affected by the neurological impact of menopause, its impact on their emotions and cognitive functioning. In addition to the 'emotional rollercoaster from hell', ADHDers named overwhelm, brain fog and memory issues as the most 'life-altering' menopause symptoms, as one participant explained:

> " 'I was good at masking and worked really hard to stay on top of things as a child, teenager, young adult, and young mother and in my working life – and I managed to cope. In my late 40s, no amount of hard work could cover up the struggles and everything got on top of me, increasing anxiety, leading to overwhelm and emotional dysregulation, and exacerbating all the struggles I had all my life.'

Difficulties controlling attention also worsened at menopause. One participant described how their unruly attentional system could no longer be forced into order:

> " 'Distractibility increased and my inability to complete work tasks in an appropriate amount of time decreased. I began spending all night working just to keep up. Things that I used to have unconscious strategies to deal with were no longer manageable.'

Across quotations, the shared experiences associated with the neurological cousins, autism and ADHD, are clear. Like autistic people we've spoken to, and as you'll hear more about in Part 3, ADHDers in the ADDitude survey describe menopause as the point where the mask broke and previous coping strategies failed. People who'd been desperately trying to hold their lives together started dropping the plates they'd been spinning as partners, parents and employees. At this point of despair, some discovered they were neurodivergent. One participant from the ADDitude survey, Margaret, wrote a more detailed account of her experiences.[30] Her life had always felt like a 'gargantuan juggling act'. Like many autistic people, she'd had a running loop in her head since childhood: 'the question, "what is wrong with me?"' Feeling as if she was 'deteriorating cognitively' to the point where she feared dementia, Margaret finally learnt about her ADHD as a result of the turmoil of menopause, which she called 'a brutal and life-changing experience'. Reaching a diagnosis through this odyssey did, however, have a positive result for some participants in the ADDitude survey, including Margaret. It meant they could receive ADHD medication, which along with HRT, helped them cope and alleviated some of these challenges.

What if you're AuDHD?

ADHD and autism commonly co-occur. One estimate suggests that 40% of autistic people also have ADHD.[31] AuDHDers (people with co-occurring autism and ADHD) seem to face struggles over and above those experienced by people with either ADHD or autism.[32] Given the commonality of the co-occurrence, we've spoken to many AuDHDers about menopause, and some of our 'autistic' experts were actually talking to us from the perspective of being AuDHDers. What were their experiences during menopause?

If we think about those two domains of ADHD features – difficulties controlling your attention, and hyperactivity/impulsivity – we can see both heightened in the accounts of our experts. Just like ADHDers in the ADDitude survey, Janet highlighted her distractibility and brain fog:

“ 'I think it is the brain issues, the brain fog that has been the hardest [at menopause]... my mind was full of everything, but I could focus on nothing. I'm so often naturally overwhelmed with thoughts and feelings, and sometimes it's positive, sometimes it's like little fireworks and light bulbs and things. But also, I very much identify with the ADHD thing of going, "oh, I'll I just go and pop that washing basket upstairs, oh that needs doing", you know, and then you sort of end up doing 100 things at once... if you add to that brain fog, it's just... it's like four times as long to get to the same point.'

While she'd previously been able to exert some control over her attention before menopause, Ann said it became 'virtually impossible' to attend to boring tasks:

“ 'It's like, squirming from the inside out. It's painful, it can make you feel very sick and nauseous, dizzy and sweaty. It is just horrible. And I didn't ever have that before... not to that point where I have to lie on the floor after it for about an hour... it feels like I've just run 18 miles just from doing maybe three hours of training, you know, because I've used every bit of my brain energy on something.'

Anne and Claire both described how their unruly attention spans affected the kinds of work they could do. Participants in our earlier research had spoken about how the 'wonderful gifts' of ADHD had turned sour at menopause, becoming highly disabling.[33] Anne, likewise, said:

❝ 'I'd always been a bit high energy... but I actually really thrived on that. Switching tasks and focusing, hyper-focusing on things, I could always do that really beautifully... But yeah, my, my focus has really changed... I've had to change the work I do, because I can't write the reports... it was making me cry, because I was just like, I've got to sit down and write this report and I just keep procrastinating and not doing it...'

The Cat talked about the hyperactive/impulsive side of ADHD, which she described as 'itchiness'. She said of her ADHD:

❝ '[It] has got way worse in all aspects. WAY worse. I feel like a lunatic, I feel like I should be sedated at all times. ADHD, good god... it [was] a walk in the park compared to what's got worse about it. I'm more impetuous and I'm aware of it, and it's almost like I'm daring myself. Impetuous, and at the same time knowing that I shouldn't be... and way more impulsive. ... That's one of the reasons I went for all the diagnoses. Because I thought, I'm getting older, I'm getting worse. I'm getting so much worse. I've got to know what the heck I am, like, there's got to be a reason for all this.'

Interestingly, both Claire and The Cat found their ADHD more difficult and impactful ('way harder work', in The Cat's words) than their autism at menopause. There is actually some suggestion from research that ADHD features may be more strongly linked to depression and anxiety than are autistic features.[34] However, it seems likely that a person's first-hand experience of autism and ADHD differs across their life course – where, perhaps, individuals who are AuDHD might find aspects of their autism more challenging at certain ages and in certain circumstances, and find their ADHD more challenging at other times.

Neurodivergent people share so much in common, from the way they experience the world to how they are treated in it. We suggest that these commonalities probably point to the need for greater support and understanding for people with other forms of neuro-divergence, in addition to autistic people, but the nature of that support might need to differ in relation to their neurodivergent pro-files. It must also hold and support other forms of marginalization and challenging experiences associated with them, as we'll go on to discuss in the next chapter.

Chapter 11

Multiply marginalized

Experiences of ethnic, sex and gender minorities

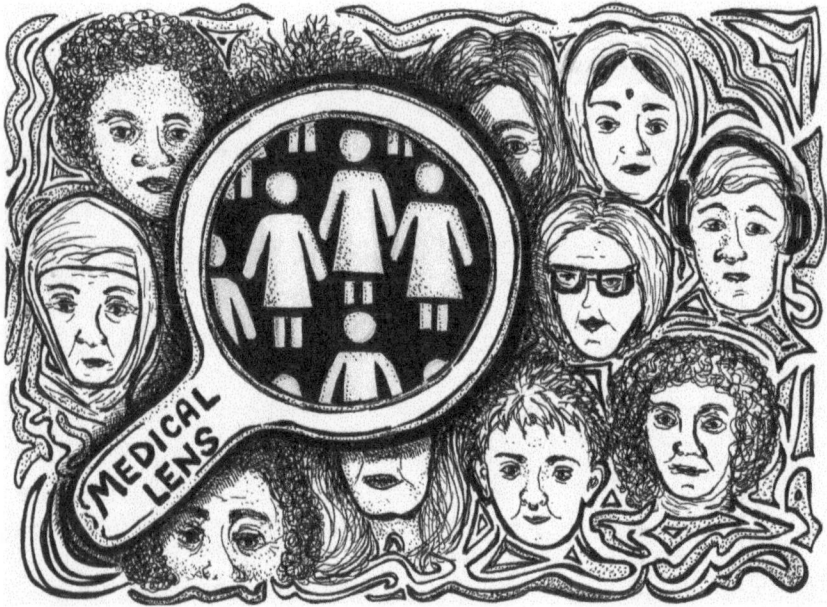

If you consult the Merriam-Webster dictionary, you'll find that inter-sectionality is defined as 'the complex, cumulative way in which the effects of multiple forms of discrimination (such as racism, sexism, and classism) combine, overlap, or intersect'.[1]

Put simply, it means that if a person has multiple characteristics which are marginalized in society, their experience will be different to that of a person with just one marginalized identity, or a different constellation of marginalized identities. These different marginal-ized identities can all have their own challenges, and sometimes when they intersect, these challenges are layered up, or the person experiences wholly new difficulties.

Autistic people experiencing menopause are already marginalized by several aspects of their identity (see Figure 11.1).

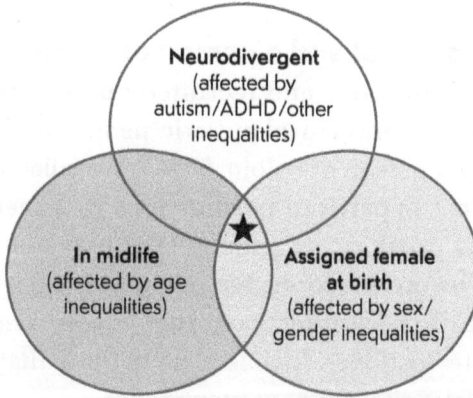

Figure 11.1 Intersectional disadvantages which might affect autistic people going through menopause

We can also see their unique intersectional disadvantage over, let's say, young autistic girls, and autistic men at midlife. Autism research and services consistently centre autistic children/teenagers[2] and people assigned male at birth,[3] so as autistic females age, they edge into that most underserved intersection. But what if, as in Figure 11.2, you're in the intersections of additional marginalized identities?

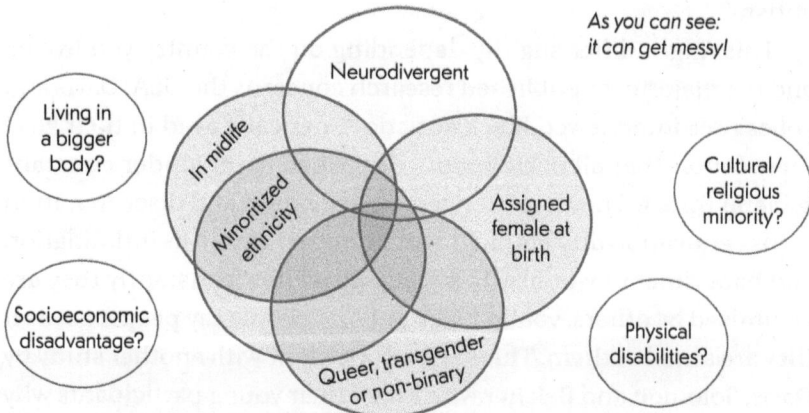

Figure 11.2 The challenges of multiple marginalized identities

There are many, many ways that a person can be socially disadvantaged or marginalized by society. We're going to consider just two of the three-way intersections that might affect someone's experience of autism and menopause: being a person of colour, and being queer.

Autistic, menopausal and a person of colour

When we began this book and recruited our autistic experts, we hoped to include menopausal autistic people who identified as Black, Brown or a person of colour (POC). We failed to recruit any, which may reflect, in part, our positionality. We benefit from white (and cisgender) privilege, so autistic POC may not have felt safe speaking with us on this topic. We recognize, indeed, that it's far from ideal for us to be writing about this, but we want to highlight the two-way intersections which lead us to think that autistic POC might have unique challenges at menopause.

Autism and ADHD occur in people of all ethnic, racial and cultural backgrounds, but educational and clinical professionals in high-income countries like the USA and UK are less likely to identify autism and ADHD in POC.[4] While this means that undiagnosed autistic POC don't have access to services, we also know that diagnosed autistic POC still experience more barriers to accessing healthcare, social, educational or employment support.[5] With research and services overwhelmingly centring and catering for white individuals, how does being Black, Brown or a POC affect someone's experience of autism?

This might differ slightly depending on the country you live in, and the majority of published research concerns the USA. Davis and colleagues interviewed Black autistic Americans aged in their 20s.[6] They found that all participants described living under constant societal threat. They experienced victimization and discrimination across education and employment contexts, as well as intimidation and harassment by police. Ironically, given how constantly they are victimized by others, young Black autistic people say people act as if they are afraid of them. This seems consistent with another study by Davis, Solomon and Belcher who asked their young participants why they thought others acted as if they were afraid of them. Thirty-eight per cent said that their Blackness was the sole reason, while 28%

attributed the prejudice to their autism alone, and 24% attributed it to being Black and autistic.[7]

To avoid this kind of intersectional disadvantage, some individuals may highlight or 'perform' certain parts of their identities over others. In another study, a young woman described being affected by stereotypes around 'angry Black women, or angry Latina women, or mentally ill Black women'. Nevertheless:

 '' 'Between the dual pressures of being Latina and between being autistic, I chose to be Latina… in many ways… identities… are based on performance, and I performed being a person of color… There aren't really visual signifiers of autism but there are of race… and it was easier to try not to be autistic than it was to not be Black.'[8]

However, others find their position in the intersection distances them from white autistic people and from non-autistic Black people. On top of the masking they might do to reduce the visibility of their autism, many POC also code-switch, adapting their clothes, make-up, language and mannerisms in order to protect themselves from discrimination when around white people.[9] One writer, explaining her difficulties segueing smoothly between white, Black, autistic and non-autistic ways of presenting herself, said:

 '' 'These differences cause me significant problems with other Black women in particular. They do not relate to me, and as a result, I experience isolation and sabotage. People reason that Black women look out for one another, but that has not been my experience.'[10]

We struggled to find published research on Black, Brown or autistic POC in the UK. What little we found corroborated that Black autistic girls similarly suffer from stereotyping of Black women as 'masculine', 'aggressive' and 'angry', stereotypes which precede recognition of any other aspects of their identity, and which get in the way of receiving support for autistic needs.[11]

While there is increasing visibility of menopause as a topic of importance in autistic people, autistic people who identify as Black, Brown or POC at menopause and midlife are still almost entirely unrepresented in the literature. This matters greatly. As we noted earlier (pages 29, 37 and 42), POC appear to enter menopause slightly earlier, may experience symptoms differently to white people, and might experience them for a longer period.[12] While this might be partially biological, it's also likely related to the minority stress and disadvantage experienced by POC in countries like the USA and UK.[13] If you think back to Chapter 4, you'll remember that a number of psychological factors affect your experience of menopause, your thoughts and feelings about it, for instance, and whether you feel well supported by friends, family and your doctor. We know that POC don't necessarily feel represented by the white narratives that are centred in mainstream media, and might have a harder time seeking healthcare.[14]

How do autistic people identifying as Black, Brown or POC – women, non-binary or transgender – experience menopause, given additional burdens of masking like code-switching, and long-term impacts of the stress associated with race- or ethnicity-related marginalization on their health? Do they feel represented by existing narratives about autistic menopause? Probably not. Until more concerted efforts are made to hear the menopausal experiences of Black, Brown and autistic POC, we simply do not know and that cannot be acceptable.

Autistic, menopausal and queer

Interestingly, there is some evidence to suggest that autistic people and ADHDers are more likely than neurotypical people to be queer.[15] 'Queer' is a reclaimed slur used collectively to describe individuals who identify as transgender or as another gender outside the binary male/female; it also includes people (cisgender or otherwise) with non-heterosexual sexualities, such as people who are gay, bisexual or pansexual, asexual and/or aromantic, or a range of other orientations.[16]

Across the world, queer people are subject to inequalities, and implicit and explicit discrimination on account of their gender and/or sexuality:[17] examples of this range from unfair treatment in higher education, healthcare, housing and employment, to legally sanctioned hate crime and imprisonment in some countries. Though menopause will affect anyone born with ovaries (including some intersex people), transgender men, people with non-binary gender identities and/or non-heterosexual sexualities (sometimes also referred to collectively as trans+ people) are rarely represented in menopause media or catered for in terms of information and support.[18] Individuals who have their ovaries removed as part of gender-affirmation treatment will be thrown into a surgical menopause, while those who retain their ovaries may enter a natural menopause around the same age as cisgender women do. For transgender men and individuals with other non-binary and/or transgender identities, menopause can be very threatening and traumatic, interfering with their expressing and living as their true gender.[19] Due to healthcare discrimination, many fear seeking help.[20]

Being queer and autistic brings with it an additional host of intersectional challenges in accessing healthcare: for example, sometimes the fact that a person is autistic is used to invalidate their expressions of their gender identity or sexuality.[21] We didn't manage to recruit any transgender men for our autistic expert group, but we previously spoke to one transgender autistic man. As someone with traumatic life experiences, he was navigating the challenges of menopause without support: 'I've gone through a huge amount in my life and almost every time I was alone. No help. Zero help. And that's very difficult... don't wish that on anybody.'[22]

We asked some of our queer autistic experts how this intersectionality had affected their experience of menopause. Florence, Spike, Lily and Anne, all expressing queer gender identities and/or sexual orientations, spoke about how they'd never really identified with common societal ideas about the female gender. Anne, who'd never felt 'particularly feminine', felt that this had protected her, to some degree, from what some women feel at menopause:

   'I don't think I have that, like, loss of femininity that maybe some women experience really profoundly... I can really see that [my friends] feel diminished in terms of their femininity, their attractiveness...like their womanhood is somehow being bleached away... Maybe it's something to do with sexuality and [the] gender spectrum, but I don't feel like my femininity has been taken away from me postmenopause.'

Lily, growing up queer in the 1970s, felt that menopause had actually resolved old issues around femininity:

" '[While growing up] I just had real problems with gender. I didn't really see myself as female. I briefly went through a period where I thought, "Oh, you know, I could be a boy"... you'd call it gender dysphoria now, I guess. And, you know, if [transitioning] had been an option, I might have thought about it, I don't know. But... I kind of felt I wasn't comfortable in my body at all. I've always felt, you know, it's almost like it was betraying me. ... I then started being attracted to women. Well, blimey... I was called all sorts of things... you get picked on because you're too autistic and then, you get your sexuality heaped on top of that. It's pretty horrendous, very, very isolating... I guess where I was going with all of that was that for me, menopause was almost like a kind of resolution of that gender tug of battle that's going on.'

Florence, in contrast, suggested that the strain of not identifying or feeling like a woman was heightened during menopause:

" 'Because I am female presenting, I've just gone with the path of least resistance and generally don't say I am non-binary... I found it hard enough how some medical professionals treated me, [so] I wasn't going to give them something else to beat me up with. But I found it harder having a woman's body during menopause... I didn't feel like a woman. Other than biologically, that is. Information about menopause was always more about my biological bits, so it didn't really cause me conflict. But menopause made me more unhappy to be a biological woman, with the strains and stresses, ups and downs of the biology. I just wanted it over.'

Spike described a greater sense of 'separation' from their body during menopause, but suggested this might have had something to do with their single status. They highlighted that with changes in their libido and 'drive' to be in a relationship, their sexuality had affected their experience less than it might have, since that side of things had just been 'left on the shelf somewhere'. Ann, who identified as asexual, expressed something similar in terms of putting aside 'that side of things'. While she'd always masked and tried to 'do what everyone else is doing' in terms of relationships, at menopause, she found herself reevaluating this approach:

> 'When I got to 40, I think I kind of thought... why am I trying to be in a relationship and trying to have a partner and trying to, you know, do all these sort of things that are expected of me, when I don't actually like it? And navigating relationships is difficult anyway, isn't it? And navigating intimacy... when you're intimate with somebody, people will say, what do you like, what do you enjoy? And I think, well, none of it really, if I'm honest. I'd rather have a nice cup of tea and some biscuits.'

We wanted to know more about the intersectional experiences of our experts when trying to seek support and access information about menopause. Spike, who described being misgendered and quizzed about their gender identity on a regular basis, said:

> 'Yeah, I don't feel particularly represented... marginalized because of being autistic, marginalized because of being genderqueer, I think you kind of come to accept that you will never be represented. So you just deal with it on your own, really... that's how it's impacted me. Feeling quite alone.'

Lily shared Spike's feelings of 'marginalization'. She reflected on the fact that two people experiencing the same thing can 'just have a completely different experience, with a different emotional reaction'. She felt that this crucial recognition was missing from support around menopause:

> 'There's so little out there, specifically in terms of healthcare for gay women, menopausal gay autistic women – well, we might as well not exist. You can't even talk to the medical profession about it, because to them, menopause is menopause... "Why should a gay woman experience menopause any differently, it's still the same thing." Same for autistic women. "It's a thing, it's a thing that you go through, and don't make a big deal out of it, it's natural, it happens to everyone and we all experience it in the same way"... so there's no information there. There's no recourse, no support, no help, there's nothing... it's just, you're just a complete invisible. You just don't exist as far as, you know, society or the medical profession

is concerned. You're just lumped into this amorphous mass of "women going through menopause".

Trauma-informed approaches are often necessary for autistic people, given their experiences in the world as stigmatized and victimized minorities. This may be even more important for those who've experienced additional layers of marginalization. Support for autistic people at menopause is unlikely to be helpful if it fails to hold and accommodate all aspects of a person's identity, as beautifully expressed in the following quote from one Black autistic adult:

> 'I am the sum of my parts, and any and all care I've received has fallen short because it's attempted to treat my parts separately if it considers them at all...
>
> Picking two [identities] is [like] unweaving the fraught, trauma-born tapestry of the person I am because I have too many colors of threads running through my story... These things are not things that accompany my personhood: they are my personhood.'[23]

In wrapping up the second part of this book, we've reviewed the numerous factors that might complicate an autistic person's experience of menopause. As you've seen, every autistic person might have a slightly different constellation of vulnerability factors – from having more severe sensory sensitivities, to reduced social support, unawareness of being autistic, other forms of neurodivergence, and/or other marginalized identities – all of which affect their experience of menopause, and all of which need to be accommodated when thinking about the support they need during menopause. Where we've been thinking about the factors that might make the menopausal experience more challenging in a theoretical way, we'll now move on to exploring in depth how autistic people experience the menopausal transition.

Part 3

AUTISTIC EXPERIENCES OF MENOPAUSE

Now we know the factors that might spell particular difficulty for autistic people during menopause, the third part of our book will delve into the experiences of our autistic experts at menopause. We'll explore the various changes they experienced and how these impacted their lives, starting each chapter with the questions we asked them and the brilliant responses they gave. We'll begin our exploration in Chapter 12, with the physical changes of menopause, followed by the emotional changes in Chapter 13, the cognitive changes in Chapter 14, the impact of menopause on their social worlds in Chapter 15, and the sensory changes of menopause in Chapter 16.

Chapter 12

Physical changes

The expected and the unexpected

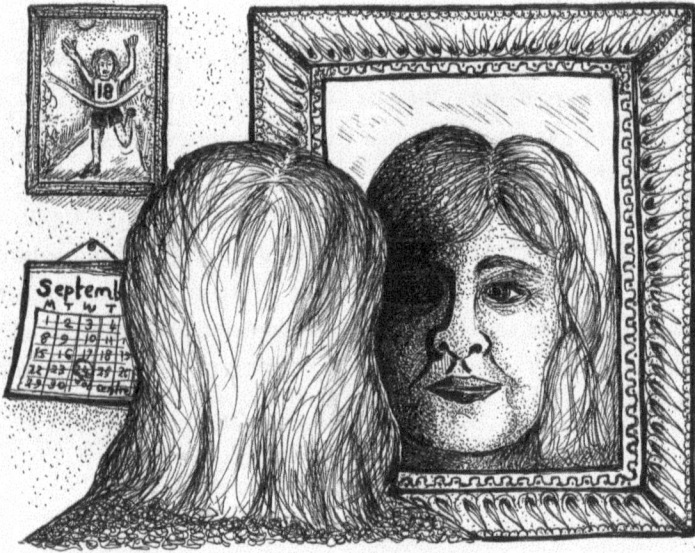

'What physical symptoms or changes did you notice during menopause?'

" 'The night sweats were horrible. I hated the sensation of waking up in the middle of the night covered in sweat. It led to me feeling very anxious at bedtime.' SPIKE

" 'I started to notice that I was having problems with my joints... and tinnitus. I never massively suffered from hot flushes.' ALICE

" 'Weight gain has been really obvious, being bloated. I've always been very fit and active. And then when you're really, really fatigued and you can't do those things, you physically can't do it, then it impacts how you feel about yourself taking on loads of weight.' ANN

" 'Heavy, heavy, heavy periods. I was having such hot flushes and nausea and dizziness to the point where I got referred to a cardiologist in case it was my heart.' BASSAI SHO

" 'Ringing in my ears, itchy skin. Irritable bowel syndrome symptoms much worse. Body odour changes. My hair's got thinner. I get facial hair, urinary incontinence around my periods, and weight gain that I can't seem to shift...' SUZI

" 'I went nuts a few times because of the sleep and the hot flushes and the sweating and the smell. You know, that my body started to smell different. Like puberty, you know, all of a sudden, my body felt like smelly and dirty. I was really worried... I [must] smell because I'm sweating all the time... My hypermobility got significantly worse, so I had really bad joint pain. Very, very difficult to exercise because my joints were really, really hurting all the time. And really extreme tiredness, almost to the point where, like, it would make me feel like I wanted to cry...' ANNE

" 'The dry skin got really bad. I would scratch myself all the time... the more stressed I got, the more I would scratch, and my skin was really sore. I was much more emotionally unstable, shall we say, in the run-up to my periods. And the constant need to have a wee.' CLAIRE

" 'My skin has got a lot drier. I can't seem to get enough moisture into it ever. My hair's a lot drier and a bit more coarse. I put on a lot of weight. I've got COPD [a lung condition] now, so therefore I find it very difficult to exercise to the right cardiac amount to help me lose weight. I used to be very, very slender, but I'm not any more – I'm rather bouncy [laughs]. Makes me feel lousy. Yeah. I hate it. It's not, it's not me at all.' BRIDIE

" 'I was clumsier, more prone to tripping. I broke my ankle badly. My pro-prioception was really poor. My hypermobility became more obvious, and gave me more aches and pains. I developed a cyst in one breast...

I also lost a couple of teeth. Hot flushes deserve a section on their own. Totally overwhelming being too hot. Wanting to take all my clothes off to relieve the heat. Under-boob soreness due to sweating and psoriasis being aggravated.' FLORENCE

66 'Not sleeping. At one point I was waking up every half an hour. Chronic fatigue ramped up. Allergies, increased hot flushes, but I didn't have them in a big way. Bone joint problems, arthritis, but I now find out I've got hypermobile Ehlers-Danlos syndrome and bone sarcoidosis as well. I think it's all connected. I have balance issues and ear issues, cystitis, bleeding, they did some investigations and found some polyps... my rashes increased, I lost teeth... and there's like loads more.' DAISY

If you think back to the wide array of symptoms that we discussed in Chapter 3, you'll see that altogether, our autistic experts experienced just about every kind. The symptoms which are often referred to as physical are a real mixed bag. They include cardiovascular and metabolic symptoms (e.g. palpitations, weight gain), joint and muscle pains and stiffness, genitourinary symptoms (e.g. vaginal dryness) and worsening chronic illnesses. Some symptoms with a neurological basis are included under physical symptoms (e.g. vasomotor symptoms, headaches, migraines and sleep disruption), while other neurological symptoms are usually classified as psychological (e.g. low mood, anxiety, irritability, cognitive problems). Going with this way of thinking, we consider physical symptoms here and then go on to think about psychological symptoms as well as communication and social changes in the following chapters.

We've found that autistic people seem to experience the same kinds of physical symptoms as non-autistic people, though some seem to find these symptoms more troubling. We don't yet know if certain symptoms are unique or more common in autistic people, or if they experience more symptoms on average. While there are (at present) only two published studies which statistically compared menopause symptoms in autistic and non-autistic people,[1] they suggest that certain symptoms, like joint pain and headache, might indeed be experienced as more bothersome by autistic people.[2] While we wait for further research to tell us more, let's explore what our autistic experts had to say on these kinds of symptoms.

Hot flushes and night sweats

As Florence said, these 'overwhelming', chiefly neurological symptoms (see page 32) deserve a section all of their own. The Cat called them 'ridiculously intense', leaving her 'absolutely drenched'. Understandably, like Spike, others of our experts dreaded vasomotor symptoms:

> 66 'I wasn't expecting them to be as bad as they were. When you get the hot flushes, it's just like a panic attack. This feeling of not being able to breathe, you know? Really oppressive. And of course, when that happens at night, sleep was just wrecked and I was tired all the time... it makes you completely irritable because you're not sleeping; it doesn't do a lot of good for your memory either. But the thing that sticks in my mind more than anything, such a feeling of constriction in your chest and not being able to breathe... massive anxiety.' LILY

> 66 'I think I stopped doing a lot of things I loved... I used to do a lot of travelling. And I just didn't want to do that any more because I just felt really out of control, you know? Because I didn't know like... "how am I going to cope if it's very hot? How am I going to cope if there's no air conditioning?" And I felt really, really self-conscious.' ANNE

Profound and unanticipated impacts of vasomotor symptoms on sleep, anxiety and self-consciousness are things we've heard, again and again, in the course of our research with autistic people. Participants in our studies spoke about how vasomotor symptoms affected their energy levels and their functioning generally.[3] Like Anne, some people stopped going out or limited their activities because they were so worried and embarrassed. Yet others, like Daisy, Tara and Alice, weren't seriously affected by vasomotor symptoms.

Period changes

We noted a lot of variation in the way periods changed during the menopausal transition. Fortunately for Spike, their periods didn't make a big song and dance out of dwindling: 'they pretty much [just] stopped... the blood is much darker in colour than before, is much lighter in quantity, and only lasts for a few days'. Others, like Suzi and Sally, found their periods got heavier at first. For some people, extremely heavy, long periods may increase risk of anaemia, which needs medical attention. We remember one autistic participant who had a very difficult time:

> 'I was wearing tampons and then back up pads... I was quite anaemic. Quite often felt very weak... I'd count on at least a week a month of really dragging myself around with no energy... at the time I was teaching... three hour classes, and so it would be break time and people would want to ask me stuff, and I had to run off to the toilet... teaching [is] quite a demanding thing for me, so I'm always quite stressed when I'm in that sort of a situation anyway...'[4]

As we mentioned in Chapter 7, problematic periods seem more common in autistic people.[5] Some autistic people we've spoken to describe pain that's immobilizing in its scale, and dysphoria that makes them seem psychotic. We vividly remember one woman's description: 'here comes the week when I can barely move, here comes the week when I'm filled with energy and really hyperactive and stuff but that's only one week of 4, and then you know you're going to crash hard the following week'.[6] Some of our autistic experts found that pain and dysphoria were heightened at menopause; others found these experiences actually diminished. However, like autistic participants in one qualitative study,[7] some of our experts pointed out that the element of unpredictability, with periods getting more irregular, was extremely challenging:

> 'With having endometriosis and my periods being very, very painful and debilitating, I would often have to plan around that... But then all of a sudden, there would be months where I didn't have a period at all, there'd be months where I had three periods... that unpredictability was really, really difficult to manage, really anxiety-making and destabilizing, just not being able to plan and not really knowing like how it's supposed to work.' ANNE

> 'I always tend to get quite definite premenstrual symptoms... Unfortunately, you can't plan anything when you don't know whether it's going to be next week or in a month. So that, that was quite... disheartening actually.

I found it just horribly disconcerting to just not know what was going on with my body from one day to the next.' JANET

Unsurprisingly, as you'll hear in Chapter 18 (page 188), our experts generally felt that the end of periods was one of the positives of going through menopause!

Weight and shape changes

Many of our autistic experts mentioned changing shape and weight during menopause, and none were particularly happy about it. Irritatingly, changes in metabolism and the distribution of body fat are part and parcel of menopause. Remember the longitudinal SWAN study we spoke about in the first chapters of this book? They found that during menopause, lean mass (the proportion of your body which is muscle, organs and water) decreased while body fat doubled, especially around the belly; postmenopause, lean mass and fat mass stabilized, but at lower and higher levels respectively than premenopause.[8] Because much of this change is due to biology rather than changes in behaviour, the additional weight is extremely difficult to shift even with diet and exercise, as Suzi, Claire and Spike all remarked:

" 'I just kept growing and growing and that I really didn't like. That really impacted on my sense of self. The fact that I just kept getting bigger and bigger.' CLAIRE

As Claire explained, it is very difficult to inhabit a body which is changing in a way beyond your control. There may be particular distress if it's changing in a way that we are taught to view as 'undesirable', and which comes with the baggage of stereotypes like 'greedy', 'lazy', 'no self-control', often seen in Western cultures like those in the UK and USA. So your body changing in this way could change the way you feel about yourself – as well as the way others treat you. In Chapter 7 (page 71), we pointed out that these kinds of changes might be especially difficult to bear if a person has a history of disordered eating and/or eating disorders, as many autistic people do, including several of our experts. Many autistic and non-autistic people living with or in recovery from eating disorders find that disordered thoughts and behaviours around eating and the body ramp up in times of particular stress, as Anne explained:

66 'Like the majority of us that have had or live with, you know, disordered eating or eating disorders, it never really goes away, does it? At times of stress or anxiety, it goes back to the body... I've always been very... controlled. So my body kind of stayed relatively the same for a very long time... quite square, quite lean. And then all of a sudden it was quite kind of fleshy and sort of feminine and round. And I hated that. I really felt very uncomfortable and self-conscious... something about the shape of my body I found disgusting, to be honest. I felt out of control. I felt like my body was... it wasn't my body. It just wasn't my body any more.'

Bridie, who described going from 'very, very slender' to 'rather bouncy', described how that related to her difficulties with ARFID (avoidant restrictive food intake disorder). People with ARFID have unusually strong, visceral reactions to the look, smell, flavour and/ or texture of foods, so they might only have a small range of 'safe' foods. Bridie said:

66 '[The weight gain] makes me feel lousy. Yeah. I hate it. It's not me at all... I haven't felt like myself for a long while. I have ARFID, I'm quite a picky eater, I got quite shamed for it by my family and in-laws, and I get quite publicly shamed, and that made me much worse with my eating disorders and my mental health... I'm now the heaviest I've ever been, and that doesn't sit well with me at all, because it does make my life very complicated and I don't like it at all.'

'Aches and pains': joints, bones, and the body unleashed

As we discussed in the beginning of this book, menopause means losing much of the protective effects of estrogen throughout the body. Stiff and painful joints, wonderfully likened to 'a baby's rattle' by Claire, affected our experts to different degrees. While some described 'aches and pains' as mildly troublesome, others described them as 'horrific' (Sally) and 'absolutely terrible' (The Cat). Several of our experts were affected by that well-known effect, thinning of the bones; some, like Florence and Daisy, suffered bad breaks and/ or lost teeth during menopause (which can reflect bone-thinning in the jaw).

As we discussed in Chapter 7, the poorer physical health of autistic people at midlife[9] is one reason why we think autistic people might have particular problems during menopause. Many autistic people we've interviewed have told us that the menopausal transition worsened their existing health conditions,[10] but ongoing research (as yet unpublished) by our doctoral student, Eunhee Kim, has allowed us to compare the health of peri- and postmenopausal autistic and non-autistic people for the first time. Of almost 1000 participants recruited, she found that autistic people were two to three times more likely to report respiratory illnesses and gastrointestinal, urinary/reproductive and neurological disorders, as well as immune, autoimmune and inflammatory disorders. What's more, they were four times more likely to report musculoskeletal disorders and chronic, complex and congenital health problems. This tallies with what we know about the prevalence of connective tissue disorders like Ehlers-Danlos syndrome and about autistic health more broadly[11] (see Chapter 7, page 74).

Almost all of our experts described navigating complex health changes at menopause. For some, there were new immune conditions, allergies, cysts and polyps, lung diseases and high cholesterol; for some, a worsening of existing hypermobility, fibromyalgia, irritable bowel syndrome, chronic pain and fatigue. For Daisy, there were multiple physical illnesses, with several of the above as well as cancer and the emergence of some rare genetic conditions. All of these play into the impact of physical symptoms at menopause, as we look at next.

The impact of physical symptoms on autistic people

Between them, our autistic experts mentioned a whole range of other changes and symptoms, like facial hair, headaches and tinnitus, as well as the impact of menopause on vaginal dryness, pain during sex, urinary leaks, incontinence and urinary tract infections. Very importantly, some experienced relatively few physical symptoms, and some commented that the psychological (neurological) impacts of menopause on their thoughts and emotions were more difficult. But what could the impact of these physical changes be on their lives and wellbeing?

You've seen the anxiety and overwhelm our experts described, the changes in how they felt about themselves, the ways some stopped participating in activities they enjoyed or needed for self-care. Almost all of them described sleep disruption and/or fatigue, in The Cat's words, 'complete and utter exhaustion'. Some found that the physical symptoms and exhaustion affected their interactions with others, while others found that intimate relationships were put under strain by genitourinary symptoms. Now, you might say that these physical symptoms aren't fun for anyone, and many non-autistic people will really suffer from them. That's true. However, we feel they have additional significance for autistic people, who often already have low self-esteem and greater vulnerability to depression and anxiety, and who can already find venturing out of the house a major challenge. Anything that 'heighten[s] the intensity of feeling different' is going to be unwelcome.[12] Lily reminded us that many autistic people are already doing extra mental work to mask:

> '[talking to people] is like putting on a performance, it always is... and when you've got in your mind that somewhere in the middle of all this, you're going to go bright red and start gasping and sweating... you think it must stand out like a beacon. And people make jokes about it... it feeds on itself and your lack of confidence and all that kind of thing.'

This range of experiences highlights how crucial it is that autistic people are supported during the menopausal transition and beyond. In the next chapter (Chapter 13), we'll go on to look at emotional changes, and consider different moods, coping, stress and distress during menopause – but we'll come back to physical symptoms again in Part 4, when our experts talk about their coping strategies (Chapter 17). In closing this chapter, we'd like to leave you with comments from Suzi, Anne and Florence, which really capture the impact of physical symptoms, and how they might be heightened by being autistic:

" 'It's probably [because of] the combination of autism and menopause [that] I feel disassociation and quite isolated... because when I'm experiencing all these physical symptoms, the sensory overload happens very quickly... I just can't participate in life with other people because I'm completely overwhelmed.' SUZI

" 'I felt quite ashamed. I felt like, at a time in my life when I should have had my life together, I didn't at all, I was just a mess. And things that maybe would have been pleasurable and enjoyable just weren't at all... I just found that my capacity and my tolerance really reduced because I was dealing with so much.' ANNE

" 'There were times I hated myself because it all felt so horrible. Perhaps worse was how some people treated me, and showed a lack of understanding. It was easier to not tell people than to get rubbish support that made me feel worse.' FLORENCE

Chapter 13

Emotional changes

Mood, coping, stress and distress

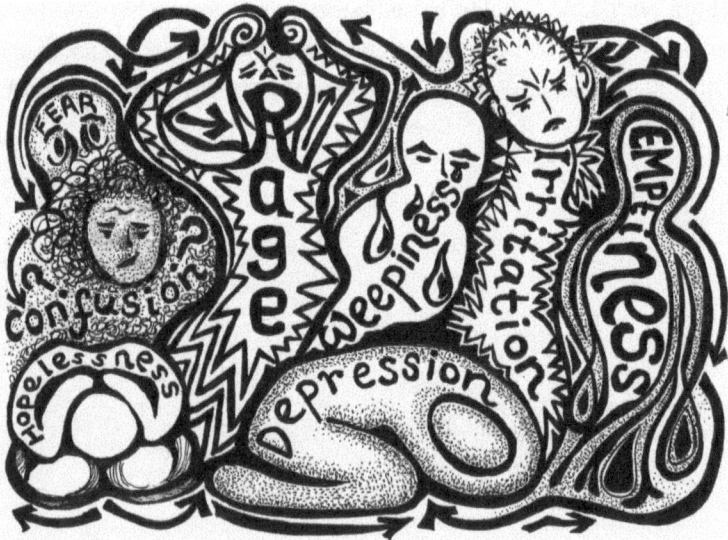

Please be aware that this chapter will include discussion of self-injury and suicide. Unfortunately, at the time of writing, there aren't any resources specific for autistic people in crisis. However, some autistic people we've spoken to have found the Samaritans (phone 116123) or the Shout service (text 85258) helpful.

If you are struggling with your mental health, with self-harm and/or suicidal thoughts, please do reach out to these or to your usual sources of support and comfort.

'During menopause, did you notice any changes to the way you experience your emotions?'

" 'It was like everything was dialled up. If it was good, it was really great. If it was bad, oh my god, it was apocalyptically awful. Anxiety was just off the scale.' LILY

" 'I would tell my family when I was feeling what I called "stabby"... they knew to tread carefully around me when I felt like that. I had ups and downs. There were times where I wished I didn't exist any more. It reminded me of puberty, only this time I knew why I was feeling like it. It didn't always help knowing, when I didn't know how to control it all.' FLORENCE

" 'All the joy seemed to be sucked out of my life... I was just so full of rage and so muddled.' SALLY

" 'Hugely. I don't think I had been overly emotional previously. I think some-times I was quite detached. But then... it was like I couldn't switch them off. I'd either be really furious or I'd be really, really sad. It was kind of out of control and it felt very scary at times because it was just a tide of stuff... [emotions] would escalate and arrive really quickly, I don't know if they would disappear as quickly, it was a bit more like a hangover...' KATIE

" 'I'm much more likely to cry at the drop of a hat, at ridiculous things... I was never really a crier before. And yeah, since the menopause started, I cry a lot more. But I feel like that's probably healthy because sometimes a good cry makes you feel better.' SUZI

" 'Going through the menopause, I definitely felt more emotionally regu-lated. But out there, on the other side, I feel more emotionally dysregu-lated.' CLAIRE

" 'This has been one of the big, huge changes... I've always been quite a weepy person... I cry if I am sad, or if I'm happy, you know, really super happy... that has always been part of my life. But just the control of it [my emotions]... they're out of control... I don't have any control.' DAISY

" 'The menopause just made me very angry. I was a very, very angry person, and I think with the loss of my mum as well didn't help because I was grieving with that for a long time.' BRIDIE

" 'Anxiety has always been a thing for most of my life... but over the past couple of years of being in menopause, serious, serious, big anxiety. But also, I never thought that depression was really part of my mental ill health. I think that I've experienced more depression in the past couple of years than I have done in most of my life.' SPIKE

" 'I get angry a lot quicker, much quicker. So that was much more difficult in my work... I found it a lot more difficult just to stay calm and be patient with people. Like I kind of lost the ability to be moderate with my response... feeling quite hijacked by my emotions.' ANNE

Our autistic experts had a lot to say about changes to their emotions during menopause. Almost all reported some change in the way they experienced their emotions and the types of emotions they experienced. Their responses also reflected the complexity of how much your menopausal experience is influenced by your psychological state and what's happening in your life. Let's explore these emotional changes more deeply in all their richness and complexity.

Changes in the experience of emotions: emotional reactivity and alexithymia

If you look at the quotations, you'll see that many of our experts reported that their emotions became larger than life; more changeable, more unruly. Psychologists sometimes speak of people having high reactivity to emotions.[1] Being highly emotionally reactive means that you:

- experience emotions very frequently and easily, in response to a wide range of situations and stimuli, like Suzi, crying 'at the drop of a hat'
- experience emotions as extremely strong and intense, like Lily with her emotions 'dialled up'
- experience emotions for longer than most other people, so it's harder to recover after being upset, like Katie, whose intense

emotions would shoot up quickly but take a long time to settle.

Given the role estrogen plays in how we perceive and respond to emotions and to possible stressors in the environment,[2] it makes sense that menopause would alter the way someone experiences their emotions. The kicker is, as we noted in Chapter 7 (page 68), that autistic people are coming from an altered emotional baseline, since many already experience their emotions as extremely intense and difficult to manage or come down from.[3]

There isn't presently any research which examines how the experience of emotion changes over time for autistic people, but by their own accounts, several of our experts seemed to become more emotionally reactive during menopause. The comments from Anne, Suzi, Lily, Florence, Alice and Daisy all suggest that during menopause, they became more sensitive to emotions, experienced them more intensely, and found it harder to recover from them. All three of these aspects of emotional reactivity are especially clear in Alice's account, which also shows how emotional reactivity could completely derail your day:

" 'These kind of emotional outbursts are becoming more frequent and harder to deal with... I think they (my emotions) are probably more intense. I'm more easily upset, so I'm more likely to cry. I'm more likely to get terribly, terribly tense. And it maybe takes me longer to recover.

It means that I will just be suddenly floored... and when I get like that, there's very little that I can do. So recently, my husband got slightly upset with me about something and I cried for 24 hours, couldn't function... I could barely coherently string a sentence together. I couldn't think straight. I just have to stop, I just have to drop everything, cancel things and take time off work... two days max and then I'm just back to normal again.'

One reason why autistic people experience emotions so intensely, and find them so difficult to recover from, is because they may only become aware of an emotion when it's already grown from an annoying, yappy chihuahua to the size and strength of an angry bear. This was clearly exemplified by participants in a study by Lewis and Stevens, who verbalized the experience of having a meltdown:

" 'For me, a meltdown is tied heavily to my emotional state. I am rarely aware of my own emotions – and I typically feel as though I am not experiencing emotion at all. During a meltdown it is as though I can suddenly feel emotion at full force, and it is such a strong, negative state of emotions that I will often lash out despite my best interest'.[4]

You might remember the concept of alexithymia from Chapter 7 (page 68), having difficulties identifying and describing your emotions. Several of our experts identified as having alexithymia; Spike, for instance, explained that they were 'OK with the general "happy", "sad" or "angry", but not so good with the more nuanced states'. Lily likewise explained that 'all my emotions are primary emotions, as it were, "good", "bad", that kind of thing'. We have previously heard from our participants that alexithymia can complicate understanding how you feel and seeking help from other people during menopause.[5] Some suggested that alexithymia might have become worse during this time, but this is yet to be explored scientifically.

Alexithymia, and emotional reactivity, also make it harder for a person to regulate their emotions. They're more likely to reach a state of emotional dysregulation, sometimes expressed in shutdowns or meltdowns. Lily, missing the finer gradients of emotion, appeared to live between the two poles of 'if it was good it was really great, and if it's bad, oh, my god, it was apocalyptically awful'. During menopause, Spike found that their ability to cope through distracting themselves was affected by their lower energy levels. Self-harm is a means through which some autistic people try to manage their emotions, and some participants told us about resorting to more frequent and serious self-harm while trying to cope during menopause. One even received a midlife diagnosis of emotionally unstable personality disorder due to her self-injury during menopause.[6] Disordered eating is also a means of changing your emotional state, which also explains why these difficulties can increase during this time of emotional instability.

Changes in the nature of emotions: anger, anxiety and depression

You'll have noticed that certain emotions loom large in the comments from our experts, such as feelings of irritation, anger and rage. Bridie explained that 'I really thought I was going mad because I was so angry all the time. I mean, *all* the time. Stupid little things like getting caught on a door handle, which happens to me frequently.' Anne described the anger 'like a volcano; I would wake up angry, no reason at all, and that was quite frightening'. Anxiety and fear, often side by side with confusion, are emotions we've heard so often expressed by menopausal people flummoxed by the cognitive and emotional changes they're experiencing: 'I thought I was going mad'. As The Cat explained, reflecting on her symptoms:

> '... you don't know *why*. And that worries you. Getting confused, more than usual. Like being confused and thinking, I don't know why I've done that... you start thinking about something and think, god, I really don't even know what I'm doing at all. Anxiety, it goes absolutely through the roof. And you just don't know why. It doesn't necessarily even have to be triggered by anything. So anxiety, depression, if you've got any of those problems, you're going to really notice it terrifyingly getting worse, especially with the perimenopause. There was a lot going on [in my family] and this was going on with me in the background and I thought, there's something really horribly wrong with me.'

Unfortunately, The Cat is correct that low mood is a prominent symptom of menopause, and an issue which may be especially worrisome for people who struggle with depression. Despite the lack of studies comparing autistic and non-autistic people, there is early indication that autistic people do indeed suffer higher rates of psychological symptoms, like depression and anxiety, during menopause.[7] Autistic people do not always experience depression as explicit feelings of sadness, as such. Some appear to experience it more as feelings of worthlessness, hopelessness, pointlessness, flatness or emptiness.[8] We heard these feelings in the comments of our experts at times, like Suzi, who berated herself for struggling during menopause: 'I just feel like I can't manage it and I should be able to, you know?' Janet explained how she oscillated between feeling too much and feeling too little:

> 'There were some days I just felt empty. But other days where all the feelings were too much. It was exhausting at times... I felt exhausted from having to, I guess, pretend emotions that I didn't feel or in the opposite hand, trying to suppress emotions that I didn't want my children to have to see or feel.'

And unfortunately, sometimes emotions during menopause take people to very, very dark places:

> 'Eventually there was the night when I couldn't stand it any more. Had a great big row with [partner], he wasn't handling it [menopause symptoms] well. I had it all planned, and I had this bag that had been packed for weeks, it had a nightdress, some brandy, letters to the kids, and the sleeping tablets of choice. And off I drove... now, I don't know what would have happened, but it was the wedding season and every bloody hotel in London, there are not many nice ones because I wasn't going to do it in a shithole, they're all booked out. And as the night wore on, I got more and more hysterical, you can imagine some woman coming in with face red with weeping, "have you got a room for the night?" [laughing]... eventually I parked the car, slept a bit, woke up and went home. And then I managed to drag myself to the doctor and say, this happened... because I'd spoken about it, I was able to carry on, because while all this was building up and building up, I hadn't said a word to anybody.' SALLY

We want to shout this from the rooftops: *no one should be so desperate at menopause that they consider ending their life.* This, if nothing else, should be as a shrieking siren to policymakers: that appropriate support during menopause, and identification of autistic people so that they can receive appropriate support, may save lives.

Autistic people are already recognized as a high-risk group for suicide, and the risk seems relatively greater in those assigned female at birth.[9] We don't know, presently, if suicide risk in these individuals changes during menopause, but suicidal thoughts and suicide attempts appeared in the stories of our research participants,[10] as well as those of our experts. We are starkly aware that though Sally was here to tell us her experience, there are missing voices in this conversation. Altogether, it plainly highlights the scale of unmet needs and the inadequacy of present services and support.

If you're struggling with these kinds of feeling during menopause, we're so sorry about this. Please do have a look at the resources we've gathered together at the back of this book, and consider reaching out to your usual sources of support and/or to the Samaritans (phone 116123) or the Shout service (text 85258) – these are both open 24/7. You might also like to look at the words of advice and encouragement from our autistic experts at the start of Chapter 17. We truly hope that things will get easier and better for you.

Emotions, menopause mindsets and the murkiness of multiple factors

Thus far, we have spoken of the emotional challenges of menopause, but you might remember Claire, whose experience appeared to go against the tide. Claire was 'more emotionally regulated during menopause and more dysregulated afterwards' (postmenopause). Let's think about this in more detail.

While going through perimenopause, Claire explained that she had escaped a bad relationship, met her new husband, completed a degree and started a new career. She said:

66 'I was more in control. I was happier, I was more contented, and I was less reactive. I was just content with life and my emotions just plateaued and I stopped having these huge dips and swings. I was now in a loving, supportive relationship. I was successful and therefore I was, you know, no longer a fuck-up; I was a nice, normal person. And that continued until I took HRT and I became angry again. I realized I wasn't necessarily maturing, I wasn't necessarily healed. I just didn't have hormones any more. And that was why my emotions kind of flatlined.'

We've heard experiences like this before. We remember one participant whose periods caused agony and intense dysphoria. She said:

'The menopause has given me a bit more confidence, because I'm the same person every day; I wake up in the morning and I've got the same mood I had yesterday.'[11]

Why do different people have such different experiences? Reflecting on our journey through this book so far, we suspect that, in Tara's words, 'there are so many moving parts'. If you think back to Chapters 4 and 5, then part of the reason may lie in the psychology of the individual, the meaning that they ascribe to menopause, what's happening in their life and how they feel about its general direction at the time. In the case of the participant we quoted in the previous paragraph, she had expressed how eager she was for menopause, so her periods would stop – if you consider her 'menopause mindset' (page 45), then for her menopause represented release from the torment of periods. In Claire's case, at the time of perimenopause, she was embarking on a new chapter, enjoying feelings of success and being in control, and well supported by her partner. The 'afterwards' of postmenopause found her in a different psychological state, where she felt much less satisfied with her life, living in a place she didn't like much, and struggling with losing her job and her sense of identity.

Undoubtedly, there are other reasons why one person's emotional experience at menopause differs from another's. However, several of our experts remarked on the fact that their emotional dysregulation at menopause could have been attributed to other things happening in their lives at the time. Bridie was grieving the loss of her mother; Spike, too, had lost a parent, and described 'huge shifts' in their life during perimenopause, including moving house and the end of a long-term relationship. Some who had new awareness of their neurodivergence during menopause also pointed out that they had new awareness of their emotional and cognitive functioning, and how that might differ from others. Tara had a very interesting reflection along these lines. She explained that she'd previously been 'really even keel, don't do big emotions'. Having lived with autistic burnout during menopause, though, and having worked on mindfulness, she remarked that although the scale of her emotions had increased over this time:

f 'I think part of that is a sort of recognition that, if I'm going to feel the positive, I've got to allow myself to feel the negative. And part of the even keel was about just numbing everything out... With all of the mindfulness work I've been doing about allowing whatever emotional state to be there and trying to take the judgement away from it, I think it's only since I've been doing more of that sort of work that my system has been allowing more emotion to come through, because I believe our systems block out a lot of stuff if it's too much for us to cope with... so have I become more emotional because of menopause-related stuff? Have I become more emotional because of distress and burnout, or because I realized that trying to mask is a recipe for nothing feeling meaningful? There's been so many other moving parts.'

In sum, so much was happening to our experts at menopause, and they were changing not only with this biological transition but also all the other many transitions and changes in their lives. While there were changes in their emotions, sometimes it was difficult or impossible to attribute these solely to menopause.

Emotion changes had wide-ranging impacts on our experts. Anne, Ann and Lily all described how emotional changes affected them in relationships, making it difficult to cope with other people. For Alice, her increased rejection dysphoria led to her increasing her efforts to please people, often at the expense of her own needs and to the detriment of honest communication. Almost all of our experts described impacts of emotion changes and menopause on their mental health.

Having looked at this array of sometimes unruly emotions, emotional reactivity and emotion regulation during menopause, we would like to finish this chapter by recognizing that some emotion changes had unexpected, hard-won silver linings. Tara's new 'great emotionality', although challenging, was a sign and perhaps a route to meaningful and authentic experiences. We have spoken to others who, through the extraordinary 'mental discombobulation'[12] of the emotions during perimenopause, reached a state of greater self-awareness, self-resilience, compassion and empathy for others suffering from mental distress. Bridie also found an unexpected silver lining to her emotional changes, saying that her decreased tolerance for 'suffering fools' led to her identifying that some individuals were 'offering nothing positive to my life' and breaking ties with them, acknowledging 'that's been quite a useful emotional regulator'.

In the next chapter (Chapter 14), we turn to the topics of attention, memory and other thought processes, and look at how menopausal changes in these types of cognitive functioning have an impact on everyday living and work. Importantly, we'll come back to emotions in Part 4, where we will look at some ways to help cope with these emotions as well as with cognitive challenges. For instance, our experts described needing to learn to be kinder to themselves, to give themselves the compassion and the creature comforts they needed while traversing this rough emotional landscape (pages 172–174).

Chapter 14

Attention, memory and other thought processes

Changes and their impact on everyday living and work

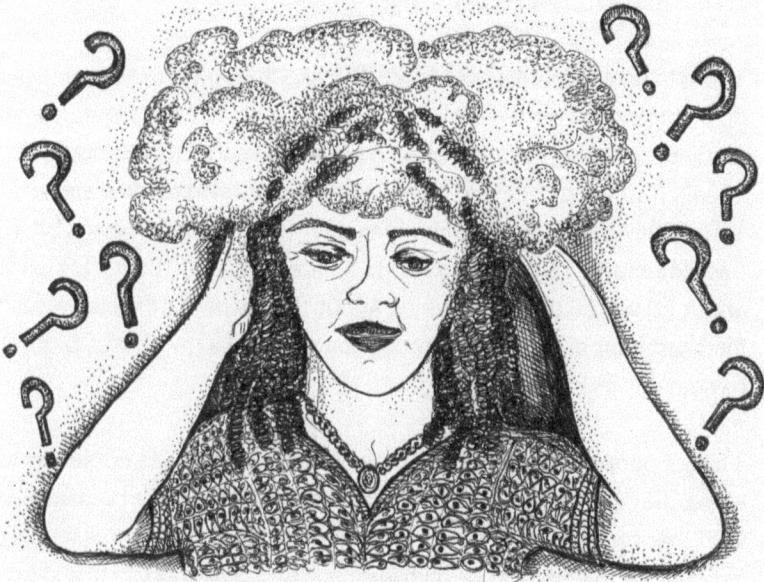

'Did you notice any changes to your memory or attention span?'

" '[I'm] feeling really lacking in energy, both mental and physical.' JANET

" 'Really, I feel quite exhausted by it. Ten years of not having my brain... I feel like I've got 25% of my brain. Occasionally I can get it really sharp again, but it takes a lot more effort now.' **DAISY**

66 'I've definitely found over this past period that my memory is not as good as it used to be... My cognitive abilities fluctuate a lot more than they used to... To what extent that's related to burnout [rather than menopause], though, I don't know.' **TARA**

66 'I started to worry I was getting early-onset dementia, just not being able to remember anything: dates, times, whole conversations, things that people had had with me, forgetting how to do really basic things on the computer, stuff like that. I thought, "this is getting a bit scary now".' **ANN**

66 'Memory has always been bad, but it's worse... I don't have the attention span I used to... It's highly frustrating.' **BASSAI SHO**

66 'I used to do a lot of crosswords, reading and that sort of thing. I can't even do a simple crossword any more, I just don't seem to have the words. And reading... it's really hard to pick up a book and read anything now, which is really frustrating because I love reading. Now, I start reading and I think, "oh no, I haven't got the attention span", my attention span is very short. The awful memory... I'll be talking and I'll suddenly forget (1) what I'm talking about, (2) what we've been talking about, (3) any part of the conversation that's just happened. I'll forget common words like my glasses or the TV remote or... it's really frustrating.' **BRIDIE**

66 'I forget people. I forget events, they just disappear. And people can say to me, they can describe to me events that they and I were both involved with that sound really memorable, like, you know, really outstanding, exceptional events. And I would just be like... no memory of that.' **ALICE**

66 'My memory and attention span have definitely changed. There are times when I can't seem to function unless I make lists and, even then, I need to remember to look at the lists, and then have the energy and motivation to execute the tasks that I've set myself. I think that's one of the big changes – my level of motivation has dropped quite dramatically. I don't feel as driven as I used to. I find it harder to get into a flow state these days and I'm more likely to struggle when it comes to switching between tasks. I've had

more mini burnouts since my periods stopped, feeling both physically and mentally exhausted to the point where I can't function like I used to.' SPIKE

" 'Memory and attention span, they both decreased. I've always ascribed it to the lack of sleep. Because when I went on the HRT and got a good night's sleep, it seemed to improve, but oh goodness. I could forget what I was saying in the middle of a sentence sometimes.' LILY

'Everyone's brain goes a bit soggy when they're going through menopause.' These words, said to Bridie by her doctor, are extremely apt. You know by now that the brain undergoes a seismic shift during menopause. A shift that feels so dramatic that Ann, like other neurodivergent people in studies,[1] feared she had early-onset dementia. Unlike in dementia, these cognitive impairments appear to ameliorate postmenopause (in non-autistic people, at least),[2] but the comparison is otherwise more relevant than you'd think. Brain imaging shows that during menopause, specifically as a result of hormonal changes rather than ageing in general, there are reductions in grey and white brain tissue across the frontal and temporal lobes, and as a result, more 'empty spaces' filled with cerebrospinal fluid.[3] As people go through the menopausal transition, their brains show greater increases of amyloid-β, a protein which is seen to build up in 'plaques' in the brains of people with Alzheimer's disease, with this effect most pronounced in those carrying one genetic risk factor for Alzheimer's.[4] While this study found evidence that the brain was adapting in postmenopausal people, who also experienced recovery of their cognitive functions, it's still sobering stuff. It is worth holding onto the fact that most people say brain fog improves postmenopause, as it does in other hormonal transition states like pregnancy and puberty, but the impact of menopausal brain fog can perhaps feel particularly worrying at the time, given we might associate it with ageing. We come back to this in Part 4 when looking at some strategies and ways to manage menopause (Chapter 17, pages 174–5).

Unfortunately, we're far from knowing if autistic brains show similar changes to non-autistic brains during menopause, but quantitative and qualitative studies tell us that autistic people can experience the cognitive changes of menopause very severely[5] and possibly to greater extents than non-autistic people.[6] This is an area where autistic people will likely share great similarities with their neurological cousins, ADHDers, who described cognitive symptoms as the most 'life-altering'.[7] Let's explore our experts' experiences.

'My brain goes blank' (Daisy): the many faces of cognitive dysfunction

Researchers have defined brain fog as 'temporary experiences of forgetfulness, cloudiness, difficulty with thinking or processing information, as well as trouble with learning'.[8] We liked Daisy's way of thinking about 'four types of brain fog'. They clearly show how multiple cognitive processes are affected, and the many consequences.

Fog type 1

> 'The one where I would sit on my computer for like a whole day and write two lines. Couldn't focus, just couldn't get my brain to unfold enough to focus on my work.'

Daisy's first type of brain fog seems most clearly related to attention. While we saw this was a major difficulty for ADHDers and AuDHDers in Chapter 11, reduced control over their attention is also a major problem for autistic folk without ADHD. If you cannot control your attention, it's difficult to impossible to get into a 'flow state', in Spike's words. Janet vividly described how distressing this is, when your work depends on achieving focus:

> 'I was having so many days when I would just sit at my computer to work and I'd just be in in tears after a while because I just couldn't, I couldn't, just couldn't do anything. There were just so many days wasted because I was getting further and further behind. I just felt constantly overwhelmed by everything.'

Attentional control is just one aspect of executive functioning, and so it relates to abilities like splitting your attention across multiple tasks (multitasking), planning, organization, stopping one thing and switching to another. These are all things that are very, very difficult to do without strong attentional control. Several of our experts expressed that multitasking, something that was challenging before, had 'just gone out the window' (Lily), that their attention could be 'easily snagged with so many things whirling around my brain, actually being able to stop and distinguish the thing I needed to do... impossible' (Katie). Bassai Sho, 'as someone who likes to be highly organized', found that the deterioration in her ability to plan was 'very, very frustrating... I just don't have the same ability that I used to be able to organize like before'. Remember, of course, that for autistic people who struggle with unpredictability, organization is really important, which is ironic since it's so difficult.

Fog type 2

" 'The one where I walk three steps and I forget. It happens many times a day. I think most people have, like, sometimes gone upstairs and then forgotten why they've gone up. But I can do it three times. Go up, okay, I've forgotten, go down and remember, okay, go up, forgotten, down again.'

Daisy's second type of brain fog is a good example of working memory, also part of executive function, which enables you to hold information in your head, avoiding distractions, so that you can meet your goals. Bridie told us that for her, it was 'complete disorder in my brain, and I find it very hard to move through it to be able to get things done.' Again, the resemblance to symptoms described by ADHDers in Chapter 10 is striking (page 104).

Fog type 3

" 'The one where I forget the word, can't find the word.'

Daisy's third type of brain fog seems related to language and memory. Word-finding problems were commonly reported by our experts, like Anne:

" 'I'd just be halfway through a sentence and I'd just be like, "I don't know where I was going with that, I don't know what the word is I'm looking for, I don't know what I'm talking about".'

Katie, similarly, said that she'd previously had 'a brain like an attic, with loads of stuff in it and I can retrieve it', until like Anne, she lost the words as she was saying them. Katie also spoke about broader language processing difficulties, where her apparent hearing problems reflected processing delays in understanding what other people had said.

Beyond word-finding challenges, our experts described many instances where their memories failed them. Suzi, who said her brain was working at 'like 60% capacity' during menopause, described her memory as 'shocking'; she explained her dependence on digital diaries, where previously she'd been able to hold appointments in her mind. Ann explained how beyond forgetting people's names, she'd forget their faces and voices, too. Face blindness, or prosopagnosia, means that a person cannot recognize even close family members. Ann said:

> 'People think I'm taking the mickey, but I can't... there's something in my brain that's not working where I recognize them. Even their voice or anything, it's just like they're a complete stranger. Very embarrassing... the last thing I would want to do is be rude... it looks like I don't even care [about people]. And that's not true, it's the opposite, really.'

Fog type 4

> 'The one where my brain just goes blank.'

Daisy's fourth type of brain fog, 'the brain blank', is difficult to pin to any one cognitive function. Indeed, these kinds of cognitive impairment defy linkage to any one domain, since as you can see, they affect so many aspects of processing. The mind 'going blank' is a very common expression of those who experience brain fog. We've had autistic participants describe it as 'fuzzy thinking' or a 'head full of cotton wool', and one who memorably explained:

> 'It's like I've become stupid... Basically, I just can't think properly, can't process information, can't remember things... I blank... when I've got the brain fog, it comes along with the tiredness, so... I'm like a zombie, I can't do what I could normally do mentally.'[9]

Several of our experts, like Spike, expressed a kind of 'mental exhaustion'. Janet expressed a sense of there being 'no space' in her brain any more, 'a whole other level of overwhelm, of everything, my brain just full like words are going to come out of my ears or something.'

Work and self-worth: 'I didn't know how much of my brain was going to turn up on a particular day' (Tara)

Cognitive symptoms of menopause affected our experts across all spheres of their lives, but one area might be especially obvious: the workplace. Cognitive symptoms are one of the major drivers of menopausal people leaving the workforce.[10] Tara, whose brain often left her in the lurch, stopped working. She said she was simply 'cognitively incapable' of doing the job. She wasn't alone. While some of our experts who'd been working were able to stay in their jobs, they often felt they were 'hanging on to life with their fingertips', in Sally's words. These quotes show just how difficult it was:

" 'I think, as an autistic woman, my self-confidence very much lives in my capacities and abilities in my mind. I've got a great memory. I'm really, really good at my job. I'm on the ball. I'm snappy, very efficient. And all of that went... I kind of lost the things where I'd found a bit of confidence in myself, you know, being intellectually quite snappy... all my coping strategies just went, because work wasn't a good coping strategy any more because I couldn't do it... I don't think I've ever felt so confused and so out of control.' ANNE

" 'I no longer felt intelligent. I don't mean to sound rude, but I was used to being good at things, intellectually.' FLORENCE

" 'I used to get so cross with myself, sort of beating myself up mentally about... "Come on, you're an intelligent woman. Why can't you do this? Why are you sitting there counting on your fingers? Why can't you remember what happened yesterday? You know how to plan, you know how to write a lesson plan, why can't you do it?"' SALLY

" '[It] dented my self-confidence and my self-esteem. Because I often berate myself, I'm very unkind to myself a lot of the time. And that just made that worse. I was constantly, "Oh, you're being stupid, you're stupid, you forgot it again," and it would make me feel like I wasn't doing a good enough job. And it made the job harder in some respects because I was forgetting things and being late; I hate, hate, hate being late. And it just made me a bit more anxious... everything was kind of running a little bit faster because I was constantly having to make up for these things that I'd forgotten.' CLAIRE

These quotes remind us of something that anyone working with autistic people should know: they are very used to feeling stupid, small, broken or deficient, so it doesn't take much to make them feel that way. As we mentioned earlier (page 91), many autistic people grow up as the square peg trying to fit into a round hole, being judged and judging themselves by neurotypical standards.[11] For many, a job or some other kind of role, achievement or intellectual pursuit provides a vital sense of being worth something after all, even if you've struggled in many other areas. To then have that taken away, during menopause, is shattering. These are sentiments that crop up again and again in studies of neurodivergent people during menopause who are devastated to be losing their skills:[12]

66 'I used to think, whatever anyone thought about me, they thought I was hardcore because I could get loads of stuff done and they were like, "I don't know how you do it" and I was like, it's easy, it really was easy, and then suddenly it wasn't easy any more.'[13]

66 'Everything I thought I was actually quite good at – completely out the window.'[14]

66 'The experience I had was very abrupt from being quite capable... to being unrecognizable as that person... being autistic can be a challenge but it does give us skills... My most noticeable thing was that I lost my skills [at menopause]... [how do others cope with] being robbed of their skills?'[15]

66 'I feel stupid, really stupid, and that's incredibly devastating to me. Because I've always relied on my intelligence, even though I've struggled with so many things...'[16]

Wider life impacts: 'It's difficult, adulting at the moment.' (Bridie)

Of course, executive function, memory, language and other cognitive functions are vital across all aspects of a person's life, including the most fundamental. Bridie explained how the 'complete disorder' of her executive functioning led to her sense of exhaustion and over-whelm in response to household tasks. This is yet another arena where autistic people can experience a sense of failure at these increasing challenges that others appear to be taking in their strides. The Cat, trying to help her son with his homework, would end up 'running myself round in circles', berating herself that she was struggling with work meant for 12-year-olds. Janet, struggling to remember all the things her children needed for school, found herself thinking, 'I'm no good at this... would they be better off without me?'

We have heard from a number of autistic people who, during menopause, experienced severe impacts of cognitive dysfunction on their self-care and daily living skills. We recall one participant who said: 'My life feels like a constant series of moving from one disaster to another, but never really fully regaining control'.[17] Here are several accounts from our participants, explaining the impact of cognitive dysfunction on their lives:[18]

> 'If I miss one day [of HRT], I become so tired and dysfunctional... within a day I feel like I can't live like this, I can't live a life in which I'm unproductive... even though it's not completely helping, it does keep me from being completely useless and I can carry on working, with a lot of work-arounds... I live with my mother, she is 82 years old, she has a lot of medical conditions but she does most of the housework, she... does many of the things that someone of my age should be doing, and, you know, I should be serving her... but I don't have the energy...'

> 'I have struggled with [executive function] most my life. But menopause has made it MUCH worse. It makes functioning normally very difficult. I am behind in so much stuff. My self care and cleaning of my clothes/flat etc has reduced practically to zero. I have... fallen into debt and other problems because of just not being able to function properly.'

Another participant described the shutdowns which arose from frequent overwhelm as 'I'd stay in bed, not be able to move, I couldn't even have my children around, I become non-verbal... I couldn't get words out, not wash, not eat, do nothing... I just stay in a dark room and totally switch off from everything.'[19]

Cognitive dysfunction has a rippling effect, impairing daily functioning; it can shake people's self-worth and make their world very small. Previous leisure activities might even be out of reach: Florence and Bridie reflected that, as formerly avid readers, they'd lost the ability to escape into a book.

Finding brain props: 'Lots and lots and lots of systems' (Alice)

Our experts often found themselves outsourcing executive function and memory to cope. While some, like Bassai Sho, received a lot of helpful support from family, others relied on paper or digital 'brains' to hold information for them, as you'll later hear about in Chapter 17. AuDHDer Alice described her strategies:

> 'So I have loads of to do lists, spreadsheets and apps... [to] keep track of what it is that I'm supposed to be doing. I write things down in lots of different formats, sometimes on paper, sometimes in an electronic form. [My autism and ADHD] are in tension with each other, but also I think they balance each other quite nicely... The ADHD makes me easily distracted, but it also means that I'm adventurous and I will try lots of different things, but the autism kind of means that I'm able to be organized because I can get so obsessed about something and be so just obsessively thorough and highly methodical... the fact that I love lists and spreadsheets and organized systems helps me to cope with, you know, things like lack of memory and being disorganized, and finding out how to keep track of things and being constantly distractible.'

Some of our experts, as we discussed in Chapter 8, ended up reorganizing their lives to accommodate their cognitive difficulties, dropping particular tasks at work, or finding new roles. Some, like Bridie, realized they'd need to build naps into their day and factor in 'two or three days when I cannot do a thing'. They were simply forced, through necessity, to slow down.

Although slowing down was a change enforced upon them, and one which had consequences for their sense of self, Spike and Lily both reflected on surprising silver linings:

" 'You kind of lose the ability to [work so hard] and start to discover that the world doesn't end if you don't do that. And so, yeah, you know, work wasn't quite so intense and that wasn't such a bad thing, actually.' **LILY**

" 'There is a plus side to this, though, in that I have a better work/life balance than before the menopause. I'm more mindful of the fact that I'm in a different phase of life now, that I'm getting older and slowing down is an OK thing to do. It feels as though navigating the transition has taken some time, and is a bit of an ongoing process.' **SPIKE**

Over the past few chapters, you might have noticed our experts touched on the impact of menopause on their relationships at multiple points. These are such an important part of our lives that they deserve their own chapter, so without further ado, let's move on to look at communication and relationships in the next chapter (Chapter 15).

Chapter 15

Communication changes and their impact on relationships

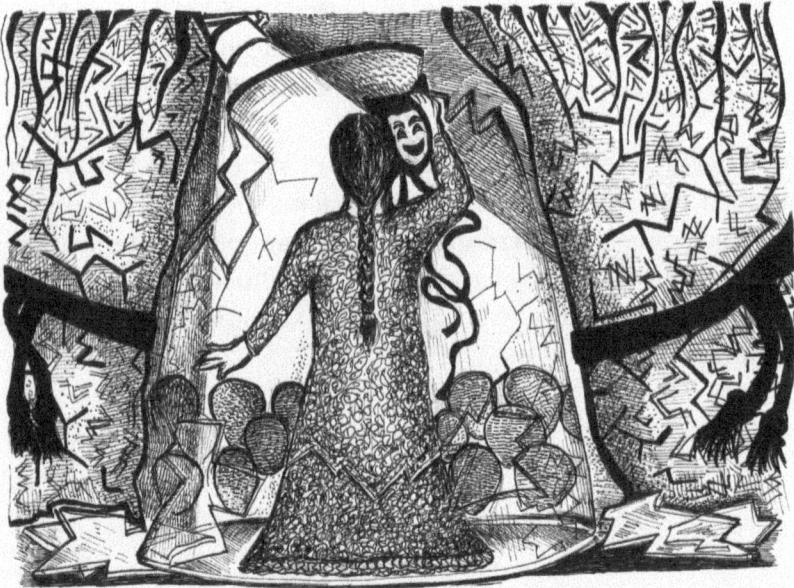

'Do you think that menopause affected the way you interact and communicate with other people?'

" 'I have always struggled with conversation, turn-taking and all that. And with the menopause, it was like... by the time I've got my thoughts in a row, it [conversation] had moved on. And so... I have nothing to contribute or no chance to contribute more, because it was all going on in my mind, but getting it down and arranged in sentences and out was... yeah. I could write it down, but I couldn't verbalize. You can hear how chopped up my speech is these days.' SALLY

66 'I'm lonely. I don't have any friends. I used to be quite good at making friends... but I'm no longer able to manage and maintain those kind of relationships. I've never been good at small talk, chit chat. But I used to be able to do it. Now I'm just blank. If I haven't got an agenda, I have no idea what to say to people.' CLAIRE

66 'I've sort of withdrawn from situations that perhaps before I could have coped with better, or that I now think might upset me – because when I get upset now or distressed about a conflict, I know it can be like anxiety for days, or even months with doctors. I know it sounds a bit harsh, but I have sort of weaned my friend group down a bit... I don't have enough energy to communicate with everybody all the time.' DAISY

66 'Because I have stepped back from activities, I feel that people, generally, have stepped back from me. I was no longer prepared to save friendships if they were too hard [work], if I felt they didn't understand. I really had to rein in any snappiness. Masking my emotions became harder. I was less tolerant of stupidity and ignorance, particularly when it came to autism, and human rights issues.' FLORENCE

66 'I ended up spending a huge amount of time on my own because I couldn't deal with other people when I was in that state and they couldn't deal with me. Kind of the best thing was to withdraw a bit and try and deal with it. I wasn't particularly able to deal with it, but at least I didn't have to deal with everybody else's reactions to it or something, you know?... A bit of an unpleasant experience, really.' LILY

66 'I think before, I was very much doing the social thing, the expected thing. But I was less able to during menopause. Maybe I didn't want to as much, but certainly, I think a lot of it was I just couldn't. I wasn't able to.' KATIE

66 'How I tend to mask is by concealing my irritation with people. I'm quite impatient, inside, but I was brought up in a very strict family and I'm extremely polite, so I would never show it. My ability to [mask] disappeared entirely. So, to people who don't know me particularly well, that

was quite a shock, I think, because it would always be "Anne's really kind, Anne's really nice". And so it sort of went from that full masked autistic woman, to somebody who'd tell you to fuck off really quickly.' ANNE

66 'I noticed that I stopped going to things. In terms of mental health, I think I detached myself from people. Like, you know, it's all a bit too much, so I'll stay home, I can manage that and feel happy. You would think that that's not good for your mental health, but for me, my mental health felt like impacted if I was trying to make myself do all those [social] things, whereas at home, I think, "oh yeah, I can cope. This is fine. I feel better".' ANN

Social interaction with non-autistic people is, in Alice's words, like a 'strange sort of social dance', and it's one that's very costly for autistic people. Negative encounters with non-autistic people are a major source of everyday unhappiness for autistic people.[1] Sadly, we know that non-autistic people do not respond well to autistic features in a conversational partner, even when they don't know the person is autistic.[2] Many autistic people try to mask their differences as a way of protecting themselves from ostracism and/or victimization, but this comes at a devastating cost for their mental health.[3] These studies show us that masking is exhausting and seems to reinforce feelings of not being good enough as you are; it can also mean that other people underestimate an autistic person's need for support.

Our experts and participants in our studies had a lot to say about what happens when these social conundrums meet with the challenges of menopause. Next, we see how it affected their social interactions and relationships.

Social communication in the time of menopause

As you can see from the quotes above, some of our experts, like Katie and Daisy, found themselves simply unable to expend energy on social interaction and masking during menopause. Many, like Daisy, Ann and Lily, found themselves withdrawing from social contact because it was so effortful, difficult and potentially harmful. Spike, who said they'd 'become a lot more of a hermit', explained that they would purposely schedule their day so as to avoid meeting others. Many of our experts explained that because they simply had to be more selective with their interactions, they had ended up breaking some of their associations:

> 'I've stopped holding onto unhealthy friendships and things like that in the last few years since I started the menopause because I'm too tired to be dealing with other people's rubbish, really. I've got enough to be dealing with myself.' SUZI

> 'I'm less inclined to take on other people's drama. I'm just like, "No, I just haven't got the spoons [capacity] to really"... And that might be just menopause, but it might also be life stresses as well. I just can't be with people a lot more than before.' SPIKE

> 'Up to five years ago, I worked standard office hours, I was in a group environment and did group meetings and all of that sort of stuff. But that sort of peopling now is absolutely exhausting. I have to really ration that... I think I've often been aware of the degree of hyper-empathy in terms of just being able to pick up other people's emotional states, and partly that's hypervigilance in terms of self-protection. I think probably I'm less able to shield myself from that now... the waves of being in the presence of another living being just hits me harder now.' TARA

Tara reflected something very profound in terms of finding herself so much more strongly affected by other people, although unable to ascertain whether that was due to her burnout or to menopause. Anne, too, had spoken about being in situations where she was 'overwhelmed' by the emotion expressed in the room and had to simply walk out, frightened about whether she could control her reaction. There is an old, profoundly damaging and dangerous myth that autistic people lack empathy. It certainly flies in the face of all the autistic people we know, and newer research is indeed now showing that autistic people are acutely, painfully, even harmfully sensitive to other people's emotions. Empathy is typically understood to comprise cognitive empathy (your ability to understand or recognize another person's emotional state based on their behaviour or expression) and emotional empathy (your ability to share another person's emotions: to be affected and upset by a loved one's pain, or to share their joy). Emotional empathy appears to be stronger, faster or more automatic than cognitive empathy in autistic people,[4] which could mean they are easily overwhelmed with emotions before their cognitive empathy can rationalize the situation. This might be especially bad if you also have alexithymia, since you might struggle to identify and even recognize where these emotions are coming from. We previously found that this pattern of emotional empathy-dominant 'empathic disequilibrium' is linked to poorer mental health in autistic people.[5] It's possible that this sensitivity to other people's emotions increases during menopause, contributing to the need to withdraw. Hopefully, future research will tell us more.

Other of our experts described how menopausal symptoms on top of other difficulties derailed their ability to communicate in the way others expected of them. Spike explained that in their multicultural city, previous difficulties understanding strong accents had grown greater ('I find it really hard to focus on what they're saying and kind of tune into their accent'). Like Sally, who struggled to formulate what she wanted to say in time to participate in conversations, Suzi said: 'I just can't participate in life with other people because I'm completely overwhelmed... I mean, even things like the ringing in your ears that you can get. I've already got misophonia and my sensory problems are quite a lot around noise. I've then got ringing in my ears as well. There's no way I can even have a conversation with another person.'

These are sentiments that we have also heard from other autistic people in the course of our research.[6] Some participants told us that with the added challenges of physical symptoms, fatigue, cognitive dysfunction, overwhelming emotions and sensory sensitivities, they found the fundamental building blocks of communication even harder. Things like picking up cues, interpreting other people's behaviour, understanding context and non-literal language, following the to-and-fro of a conversation, especially in noisy settings. We recall one participant who struggled so much during menopause that she compared it to a sub-optimal state of illness: 'My body was not a normal state. How can I be expected to, to act normal when I have to manage that much stuff?'[7] This participant often lost her speech when overwhelmed or distressed, saying that she could only groan, scream or cry. She said that during the exhaustion and overwhelm of menopause:

" 'I would lose my ability to communicate properly on, on multiple levels... so then I would have to start trading off [what] I'm going to preserve. So first thing I would lose would be eye contact, because then I knew I could still focus on the content and I could focus on the tone of voice, but it would be difficult to maintain the body language... [but] my colleague would get angry with me because I'm no longer making eye contact... [but] then if I focused on the eye contact, then I couldn't focus on the content any more. So, then I could try to get the tone right, but I would be talking nonsense. Um, so if I would eventually lose the eye contact, I'd lose the body language and the next thing would go would be tone. I would try to focus on the content but then my tone would turn, uh, trying to keep it nuanced so it didn't go bland, would mean that at attempting to put in tone, I would overdo it, so it started to sound pedantic...'[8]

We've spoken to a number of people who found that alexithymia got in the way of their being able to explain what was happening to them and seek support.[9] Our participants sometimes found that doctors underestimated their distress because they weren't crying, or would 'completely misunderstand' what they were trying to say because their emotional state wasn't what the doctor expected. Lily, likewise, said that alexithymia made it difficult for her to express what was happening for her, and the attitudes of other people were immensely frustrating:

" 'I was trying to come to terms with what on earth was going on with me, and I was trying to communicate that to people... there was no real way of communicating what the heck it was, you know, except, you know, I don't feel good, which is not very helpful to people, really... and all I could really ascribe it to was menopause and then that led to people saying, "you're massively overreacting, why are you overreacting?" I couldn't deal with that because I felt that they were trivializing what I was going through with no understanding, or not wanting to understand.'

Giving yourself space from other people is an essential and very valid autistic coping skill, as we'll discuss in Chapter 17 (page 175). It's very different, though, when this is not by choice.

Some of our experts felt deeply disconnected and left behind by these difficulties communicating. Sally, for instance, expressed how it tapped into her worsening self-image. She told us about a story she identified with, where the female character is 'pushed away, shoved on a shelf, everyone has kind of moved on and they're in the next room now'. While she'd previously been part of social activities, she now felt 'middle-aged, sidelined, unattractive, unheard'.

Menopausal unmasking

Not all of our experts engaged in masking, but many did, and reflected on the person they'd been before menopause, or the person they'd expressed and thought they were. 'Nice and kind Anne' was 'quite placid and passive and would go along' with things, like Katie, who 'did the expected [social] thing'. Suzi 'really [tried] to make everything safe and comfortable for everybody else and not think about my own needs', and Janet explained that it was becoming harder and harder to be 'that kind of super organized person I pretended to be'. Bridie 'was always a peacemaker and diplomatic in the past, anything for a quiet life really – that's how I had grown up, understanding that that was the way I needed to be'. She'd forced herself to go to all these social events she hated, much like Ann, who used to be the life of the party but who was now very withdrawn if forced to attend. Ann said:

> 'I don't understand it because I think, how could I have been such a social butterfly, who's the main person in the group of people and it was fine, and now it's not. I don't understand that, I've not worked that out. But then I thought, well maybe I was like pretending I was like that and again, over-compensating maybe. You know, "Ann's the fun one, you know, she's very loud and she's very funny and she tells all the jokes," but maybe I was sort of, I wasn't really like that anyway. Because I couldn't manage it, I *became* that and then I could go home and go phew, you know, done it.'

If you think back to Chapter 9 (page 90), you'll remember that masking is a very common experience for autistic people assigned female at birth, and especially those who were undiagnosed as children. There are many ways that autistic people mask. Cook and colleagues[10] asked autistic people all the different ways that they masked, and came up with a list. What Anne, Suzi, Bridie and Janet seemed to be describing was termed 'innocuous engagement'.[11] It's not specific to autistic people, but seems related to anxiety and possibly even social trauma, and involves people-pleasing, deferring to others, seeking approval, apologizing, centring the other person and their needs, and avoiding being in any way problematic, confrontational or too much. Ann's description also has something of appealing to others in it, and she also described using alcohol to help her 'perform' this fun persona.

Fascinatingly, during menopause, our experts and the participants in our research often found the mask slipping or breaking. Some found themselves tossing it aside. While for some, unmasking was unintentional and beyond their control, many found that there was at least some degree of intentionality in unmasking, even if it was only because they'd realized the consequences of unmasking were outweighed by the increasing cost of doing it. We explicitly asked our experts whether they found themselves less able or less inclined to mask during menopause. Their comments were so insightful that we'd like to give you them in full!

" 'I don't see why I should do to be honest. I've never been a big fan of doing it, masking. It's just something that you're just brought up to do... I'm actually at the point where I won't do it. If I feel like being a bit silly and a bit flamboyant, I'll do it. I've said this before and I'll say it again, if you don't want me to disco dance in Asda, don't put Sister Sledge on over the Tannoy.' **THE CAT**

" 'Yeah, I'm becoming less bothered, really... I make less apologies. And I'm less bothered about my idiosyncrasies now. Because I don't always notice social cues or the things people say to me, it probably affects other people more than it affects me because I care less so I notice less... If they don't want their life enriched by us autistic people and difference and how we are, then they're not the sort of people I want to be around.' **SUZI**

" 'Because I was so anxious and so irritable and such a lack of sleep, my ability to do that was greatly diminished. And frankly, I just, at that point, people were irritating me so much, I didn't care. So, yes, my willingness to do it really dropped off.' **LILY**

" 'In some ways, [unmasking] is profoundly liberating, but I think when you're not doing it deliberately, just feels a bit frightening, and you go home and replay conversations and think, "I really wish I hadn't said that"... I think I'm in a place now of being assertive, whereas I think during menopause it was just anger... I wouldn't have a choice [how I responded].' ANNE

There is a real mix of the positive and negative in these experiences: while there's joy and freedom in The Cat's dancing in Asda and Suzi's choosing to retain relationships with people who appreciate neurodiversity, it's also clear that Anne's and Lily's unmasking did not occur entirely through choice but in relation to raging emotions and exhaustion.

For some of our experts, dropping the mask was quite clearly linked to their realization of their autism rather than necessarily their menopause, although the two came hand in hand. Interestingly, these individuals tended to reflect more positive attitudes about this unmasking, which is consistent with the way people typically describe an autism realization as positive in the overall scheme of their lives (page 94):

" 'So it's both the ability but also the intention to do it. I think that since I became diagnosed, I feel like "why should I mask like I used to?"... I do still do it, depending on who I'm with and where I am, but I feel more comfortable now with being me, and saying, "actually being me and being neurodiverse is actually not a bad thing"... the diagnosis, it's given me a lot of freedom, a lot of empowerment, actually.' DAISY

" 'Now I know that I am autistic, I find, even autonomously, I can't really mask, I don't have any huge desire to, and I also find it, the mask, just doesn't want to go back on. I have no filter now... Now that I understand that I'm autistic, I feel a lot freer to be expressive of who and what I actually am. I think the menopause didn't affect it, but knowing I'm autistic did.' BRIDIE

" 'Realizing that I could be autistic came sort of like part way [through menopause]... there was a lot of thinking, "who am I?", and I started to realize that, perhaps, the person that I sort of portrayed or tried to be or thought I should be, wasn't quite me. And it became so much harder... to sort of put on that face... I'm still very much working through this. The way I dressed changed quite significantly. I realized how uncomfortable a lot of things made me, and I suddenly discovered a love for pure cotton elasticated trousers and bright colours... I think some of that was almost like, a sort of subconscious visual thing that I was doing to go along with the "OK I'm not quite who you think I am." Just small little things that I just started to do, which felt more like, just me going with me... the clothes, and occasionally sneaking into conversations about Rubik's Cubes and mini beasts and stuff like that.' JANET

66 'Since getting my diagnosis, I have thought, well, "why bother masking?" I mean, I've masked all my life and it's made no difference in my ability to get people to like me. So I might as well just give them the full me and not waste energy masking.' BASSAI SHO

It's often hard to tell how much unmasking is due to menopause or due to that increased self-understanding and with it self-acceptance, recognizing yourself as a 'brilliant, beautifully functioning zebra' rather than a 'broken horse', in the words of one of our participants.[12] This blossoming and unfurling was generally experienced as a positive thing by most of our experts, as you'll hear more about in Chapter 18, though for some, there was an element of lost control.

Menopause as a time of social and self transformation

As you can see, menopause is a time of social change for autistic people, and not all of our experts' relationships with friends, family and romantic partners survived the new unmasking and radical honesty. In part because they needed to be more selective with their limited social energy, many of our experts described some kind of streamlining of their relationships to keep only those which were meaningful and reciprocal, with people who shared their values. Anne explained that menopause was 'transformative' and had 'galvanized' those relationships that still existed: 'if it survived that it'll survive anything, right, if you've got two menopausal women and they can still be friends postmenopause'.

It is also a time of self-change, partly due to the realization of neurodivergent identities. Not all of our experts were happy with the way their social and private selves transformed, while others, like those in our research, described finding a greater sense of authenticity and self-peace at the end of the process.

In this chapter we've looked in depth at communication changes and their impact on relationships during menopause. Our experts have very clearly illustrated that menopause affected their social communication and the way they interacted with people. This was particularly so with regard to masking: while it became more difficult during menopause, there was a very definite feeling postmenopause of caring less about having to mask, and this was often a positive and liberating thing! They also described a mix of positive as well as negative aspects of self-transformation and identity around menopause. In the next chapter (Chapter 16), we take a look at another very important part of the autistic experience: sensory differences and their impact at menopause.

Chapter 16

Sensory changes and their impact at menopause

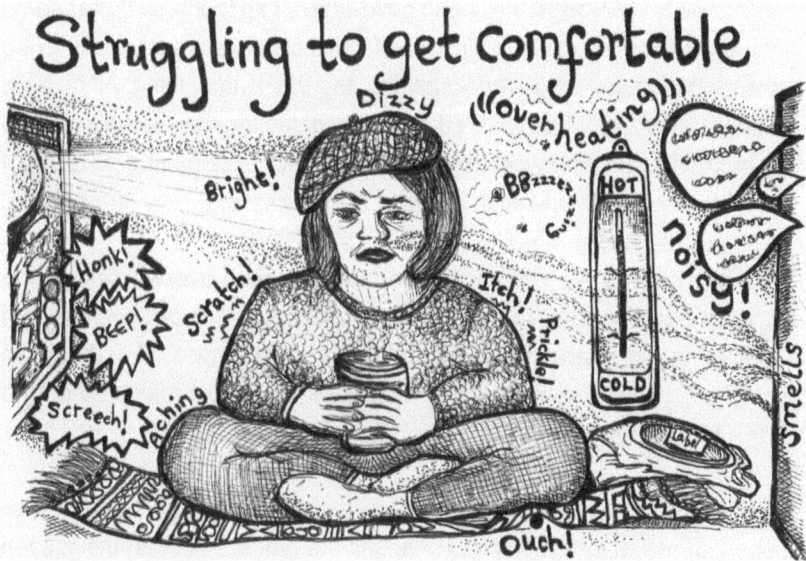

'Did the way you experience your senses change during menopause?'

" 'I used to be able to focus in, I used to be able to select, if I was in like the pub or a large room, I could focus in on a particular conversation. Now I can't do that. It's all just a great big cacophony of noise and I can't hear even the person sitting next to me.' CLAIRE

" 'It all escalated, sensitivity to noise in particular... even the slightest little noise would be like... it would go through my body. There are certain noises like drilling which have always been like that for me, but it was everything. Like the way the cat meowed, television being on one setting higher than it usually is... I would just be like, I just can't tolerate it. The feeling of things on my body... it's like using up a lot of my capacity, just tolerating, having clothing, touching my skin. Having a shower is much more difficult... I've always loved being in water... but even just the feeling of like the water on my head when I was washing my hair, I just found it really uncomfortable.' ANNE

" 'I'm sensitive to sound. The more tired I get, the worse it gets. If I come to the end of my energy, it sounds really oppressive, and there's misophonia and tinnitus in amongst that. I also have issues with touch, so there's some things, I can't even think of... I'm one of these classic autistic people taking the clothing tags out of all my clothing and that kind of thing. All of these things get worse when I'm tired or when I'm feeling quite emotional... so those things became worse because of the lack of sleep and because of the anxiety attacks and all that kind of thing.' LILY

" 'I began to find shopping centres and supermarkets overwhelming – the combination of light, sound, colour, chaos, choice is overwhelming. I passed out in supermarkets several times – was carted off to A&E with anxious children on at least four occasions. This effect mitigated during HRT. Post HRT it returned.' SALLY

" 'Some things have intensified and other things have kind of dulled or lessened. Sense of taste, I have to over-salt the hell out of everything, even more now than I ever did because I can't taste anything really. My sense of smell is intensified to the point where I can smell people making bacon sandwiches when there isn't a smell at all. My hearing's intensified... I'm more sensitive to noise. I get more annoyed, I get more short fuse... I can tolerate strobe light more than I used to be able. But bright lights, no, way worse.' THE CAT

" 'Most of my senses were affected. I struggled much more with unpleasant or overpowering smells. I became incredibly hearing sensitive, seeking quietness and solitude. Touch, fabric materials became so much more important. I would buy four of the same item so that I had enough.'

" 'My mum always used to call me the princess and the pea – you know
the story, where the princess can feel the pea through all the mattresses,
because I'd be able to feel one tiny little hair or whatever tickling my skin.
So that's even more, now, I'm hypervigilant with that even more so. Can't
bear anything around my neck. Didn't used to be too much of an issue.'
BRIDIE

Touch, taste, smell, sound and vision. Each of these senses or sensory modalities cropped up in our autistic experts' accounts of menopause. Some people found that multiple senses were affected, or just one or two. For some, their sensory experiences were heightened and for others like The Cat, certain senses seemed blunted. Our autistic experts also differed in how severely they were affected by sensory changes during the menopausal transition. Sally spoke of her frightening experiences passing out in the supermarket, but we've spoken to others who said they didn't really notice any changes in their sensory experience.

There's so much variety here, which leads to many questions about why autistic people differ so much in how they experience their senses, and why sensory changes manifest differently at menopause. We don't have all the answers to these questions yet. Let us think about autistic sensory experiences a bit more deeply and explore them in a lifespan context, so we can understand why they might change during menopause.

The variety and impact of sensory differences in autistic people

Not all autistic people have atypical sensory experiences, but studies suggest that anywhere between 74% and 95% do.[1] The sensory differences that affect autistic people and ADHDers tend to be categorized into three types:

- **Hyposensitivity**: being under-sensitive to sensations. You might not notice someone touching you or calling your name;

you might, like The Cat, overdo it on the spices and condiments on your food, not picking up the flavours until they're really strong.

- **Hypersensitivity**: being over-sensitive to sensations. You might find certain noises painful and distressing, or that certain types of light or a flickering bulb make you feel sick, dizzy or overwhelmed. You might, like Bridie, be like the fairy-tale princess, hyper-aware of a bump, lump or scratchy bit of texture.

- **Sensory-seeking**: You might find that you're fascinated or get great pleasure from the way something sounds, moves, looks, feels, tastes or smells; you might have words you love to say and hear, might love fairy lights, fireworks, spinning objects or rollercoasters.

It gets much more complicated, though. Like The Cat demonstrated, people can be hypersensitive in one sense and hyposensitive in another. You can also be hyper- or hyposensitive at different levels of processing. For instance, it's possible to have extreme emotional reactions to sensory stimuli, such as sounds, even if brain scans and hearing tests show that you're not especially sensitive to sounds at a physiological and perceptual level.[2] People can also struggle with sensory integration, like Sally in the example above. This means that it's difficult to make sense of all the information that's bombarding your senses.

For some people, differences in their sensory experiences might not be very noticeable, since we can't easily compare our own inner experiences to those of other people. For others, sensory differences are severely debilitating, affecting their sleep, the clothes they can wear, the food they can eat, the places they can go, the things they can do, and how easily they can communicate and connect with others, including in romantic relationships.[3]

Sensory hypersensitivity, in particular, has been strongly linked with poorer quality of life and greater anxiety in autistic people.[4] Autistic people say that sensory overwhelm can temporarily paralyse them and prevent communication or coherent thought, and it can feel like their senses are 'under attack'[5] every single day.

Reproductive hormones and the senses

Now, you would not immediately think that reproductive transitions like menopause would affect your sense of sight, touch, taste and so forth. If you think back to the involvement of sex hormones in emotion and thought processes, though, it starts to make just as much sense, since they affect brain-based senses, too. Interesting fact: did you know, there are even estrogen receptors in your ears?[6]

Although sensory changes don't tend to feature much among the rich variety of menopause symptoms described by non-autistic people,[7] we know that the sensitivity of the auditory, visual and olfactory systems are affected by monthly menstrual hormonal fluctuations.[8] Most research appears to focus on hearing and studies seem to suggest that in people assigned female at birth, hearing is most sensitive during times where estrogen is relatively high.[9] Accordingly, there is loss of hearing sensitivity at menopause, when sex hormones dip. During pregnancy, when estrogen and progesterone are high, effects such as tinnitus, changes in ear pressure, and greater sensitivity to certain frequencies can occur. The picture seems rather more complicated for the other senses, but they too appear to be affected by reproductive transitions like pregnancy and menopause.[10]

So what about autistic people, already neurologically different and many experiencing unusual sensory phenomena? You might remember, back in Chapter 7 (page 73), that we spoke about the heightening of sensory challenges during periods and pregnancy, with greater risk of meltdowns and overload. It stands to reason that we might see something similar at menopause, too.

Autistic people's menopausal sensory experiences

Our autistic experts clearly demonstrated that the menopausal transition affected their sensory experiences, but to different degrees. Several of our experts described avoiding crowded, loud spaces, or being driven from the room, at home, by the sound of the TV. Bridie and Anne both talked about changing the clothes they wore, being unable to stand certain fabrics or textures against certain body parts.

Sensory hypersensitivity at menopause is something we've heard a lot about in the course of our research. Participants we spoke to reported very similar impacts of heightened sensitivities on their lives, but we remember one AuDHD woman, undiagnosed at the start of menopause, who described these sensory changes as 'a major dominating, incredible, awful, debilitating thing'.[11] She gave us many more helpful insights into the many possible impacts of heightened sensitivities at menopause:

> 'Sensory overload was that bad I didn't always want to leave the house... after my sensory overload was effectively treated, I still had a mild post-traumatic stress from that period, so I had a fear of supermarkets... sometimes my food supplies would start dwindling at home and then supper might be eating peanut butter off a spoon...'

> 'It became difficult for me to take care of myself because I couldn't handle visual clutter, so I couldn't tidy... there was one stage when my mother... she came over to my flat, I lay on the couch while she washed my dishes, she helped me to fold the laundry, I couldn't do this myself, I was in sensory overload. I was exhausted.'[12]

Heightened sensory sensitivity appeared to touch every aspect of her life, including intimate relationships:

> 'If I was touched in a sexual way, like I was touched on my inner thighs for example, it was a terrible feeling... I thought there was something wrong with the relationship, I thought, "I thought I loved him, why don't I love being touched by him"... actually it was primarily sensory... I didn't have words for the sensory feelings, I didn't know that they existed... Even after I had discovered I was autistic... even when I had that knowledge and I had that vocabulary, sexual touch was very, very difficult... I would lie there tightening up because now a hand is going to touch onto a breast and it's going to hurt and it's going to be awful and everything.'[13]

Sensory mess – the complexity of sensory sensitivities

Now, if you're someone who likes to understand the biological underpinnings of these phenomena, as many autistic people do, you might have noticed something odd in our descriptions above. We mentioned how hearing, in particular, seems to be most sensitive in people assigned female at birth when estrogen is at its highest. But we also spoke about how autistic people seem to have heightened sensory sensitivities during times when estrogen is low (during menopause, and just before and during monthly periods), as well as during times like pregnancy when estrogen and progesterone are very high. It doesn't seem to quite match up, does it? Are autistic people unique, or is something else going on?

This is a conundrum to which there is currently no clear answer, but our autistic experts recognized that heightened sensory sensitivities at menopause might have a number of explanations:

❝ 'All of these things get worse when I'm tired or when I'm feeling quite emotional… so those things became worse because of the lack of sleep and because of the anxiety attacks and all that kind of thing.' LILY

❝ 'In terms of the sensory stuff, as with everything, it's very difficult for me to parse apart what is menopause, what is ageing, what is burnout… I'm remembering how much tension I was holding in my body… I'd be having tension headaches, I'd be throwing up because of the tension and would not be aware of the degree of tension I was holding in my body.' TARA

Lily's comment reflects something fundamental about the brain. Thought processes, emotional processes and sensory processes are very much interrelated, and to some degree, they draw on the same brain circuits. When we experience stress, a process which, if you remember back to Chapters 4 and 5 (pages 48–52 in particular), involves cognitive appraisal of a situation (e.g. 'Am I in control of this situation? Am I being negatively evaluated by others?'), it kicks into action a physiological and emotional response. This complex chemical reaction can actually result in sensitization of the auditory system, and this can instigate a vicious cycle where a person is more affected by and aware of sounds, which further sensitizes and, if prolonged, potentially damages the auditory system.[14]

Accounts from autistic people support that when they're under strain or struggling with unpredictability and lack of control, their sensory sensitivities are heightened, which further increases their stress.[15] Sleep disruption, too, appears to heighten sensory sensitivities while being worsened by the same.[16] Of course, stress also interferes with sleep, and sleeplessness affects how reactive you are to stress.

We can't really separate out the tangled relationships between sensory sensitivity, stress and sleep, but it's very clear that times of heightened sensory sensitivities in autistic people (around pregnancy and menopause) are times of heightened stress and sleep disruption. Another state of exhaustion and heightened stress reactivity is burnout: a state sometimes caused by sensory overload and which, unfortunately, likewise heightens sensory sensitivities.[17] It makes complete sense that Tara wouldn't have been able to differentiate the sensory effects of menopause from those of burnout, which happened around the same time.

Several of our experts pointed out another factor which might partly explain changes in their sensory experiences at menopause: the fact that menopause coincided with realization of their autism.

66 'This is, again, where things get a little bit tangled... it gets hard to separate the journeys, if you like. I am aware that I have become more attuned to sensory things, but I can't be sure exactly what is causing what... I think it's too intrinsically linked in with my autistic journey, if that makes any sense.' JANET

66 'Yeah, how I experience my senses has changed... lights and noises are more prominent in my life now. But whether it's that I've become more aware of them or it's actually changed, you know, it's [probably] a bit of both. I know now that I really, really struggle with noisy places and background noise... when I was younger I might have gone to a pub just to be sociable. I don't do that now... but whether that's sort of acknowledgement of something that I already struggled with, I'm just now more aware of it so I don't do it, or whether it actually has become more, you know, more prominent...' DAISY

Just like our participant, Janet and Daisy realized that they'd only recently had the language of sensory sensitivities and the knowledge framework of autism to make sense of their experiences. As such, they might have been noticing sensory differences far more.

None of this is to say that menopausal sensory challenges are not real, or that they are not impactful. Our experts and our research participants show just how profoundly impactful they are. It's just to show how complicated sensory experiences are, described as a 'big spider web of things' in one study.[18]

Because they are so individual, and so complex, it's difficult to suggest coping strategies for sensory sensitivities during menopause. Autistic people we've spoken to have taken very individual approaches, which centre around avoiding sensory triggers (like Florence, who 'picks and chooses' where they go), reducing or mitigating the impact of unavoidable sensory triggers (like Anne, who needed noise-cancelling headphones for the first time, or others who plan in 'recovery time'), or seeking helpful sensations to counterbalance the harmful ones (like Spike, who had an impressive array of fidget toys). We hope one day that there might be a list of ideas for sensory coping during menopause, which would be a fantastic resource for future generations.

In this chapter we have looked at sensory changes and their impact at menopause and have seen a variety of individual sensory experiences for different people as well as an increased cumulative sensory experience. We discussed how reproductive hormones influence the senses, and how sensory sensitivities at menopause are particularly important and complex for autistic people. Having covered multiple aspects of the menopausal experience for autistic people, from their physical symptoms to their emotions, thought processes and communication, we embark on the fourth part of this book, where we focus on managing menopause. We begin in Chapter 17 with advice from our autistic experts about how to navigate menopause.

Part 4

MANAGING MENOPAUSE

In the last part of our book, we hope that readers will find information about coping with menopause. In Chapter 17, we present words of advice and encouragement from our experts to autistic people approaching or going through menopause right now. Because knowing that there may be better things on the horizon, that it won't last forever and how things might change in the future are important aspects of coping, we first explore the positives that our experts found in traversing menopause (Chapter 18). Then we ask them to tell us about their experiences of life on the other side, in postmenopause (Chapter 19). Finally, in Chapter 20, we'll explore our experts' advice for healthcare and other professionals with a key role in supporting autistic people through menopause, offering insights which we hope will also help autistic people and those who support them to advocate for better care.

Chapter 17

Autistic experts

'Advice for autistic people about navigating menopause?'

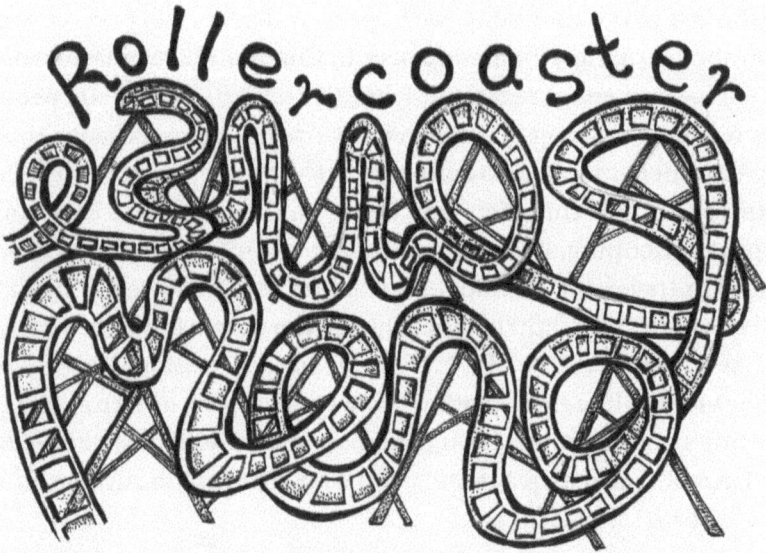

One question we asked our autistic experts was what advice or words of encouragement they could offer autistic people who were approaching or going through menopause. They gave us some really insightful answers, as you'll see here.

Be prepared
Although the menopausal experience differs for everyone, our autistic experts agreed that it can be a turbulent time, during which autistic characteristics may become heightened and existing health

conditions exacerbated, just as research has shown us.[1] Thinking back to that very apt rollercoaster ride metaphor for menopause used in earlier chapters, many of our autistic experts described needing to be prepared for what might be a 'bumpy ride':

> 'It's a massive transition. So yeah, be prepared for a bit of a bumpy ride. It's really hard, though, because [you] don't know when it's going to start and you don't know when it's going to end. And the uncertainty of it... it is so unique and so different for everyone. I mean, you've met one autistic person, you've met one autistic person. I think that's probably the same with the menopause as well. You've met one person who's gone through the menopause, you've met one person who's gone through the menopause. I think it impacts people in different ways and life circumstances can have an impact as well. You know, I'm self-employed and single and live alone. So my experience of menopause is going to be different to someone who's married with kids and who's got a regular job.' **SPIKE**

Others advised to be prepared by watching out for subtle changes and being mindful of symptoms that might indicate that perimenopause is soon to begin. As The Cat advised any woman or person assigned female at birth, 'once you get into your late 30s, maybe 37, keep an eye on it. Look out for that sweat... feeling completely exhausted for no reason at all. I mean exhausted to the point of "I ain't going nowhere," "I can't do this." And I would say to them, "You're going to start getting forgetful. Look out for that."'

Remember it won't last forever

Importantly, our autistic experts insisted that despite how it may feel at the time, and despite the rollercoaster-like twists and turns, it's important to 'just try and hold on' (Bridie), since the menopausal transition will at some point come to an end. When it does, the landscape may even look and feel calmer than it did before menopause:

> 'It will end. It will end. It's a process, and like puberty, it will end. When you're in it, it's really difficult to know that. It's really difficult to feel like there's any ending to it all because it just feels so awful. But it does end...

You will come out the other end and you probably feel better than you did before. There is light at the end of the tunnel. Yes, it's all right.' ANNE

" 'Life does get better. Yeah, it really does get better, because periods and things like that are so triggering and so overwhelming for [a lot of] autistic people... so that's great, being on the other side now, you're not going to have all these hormones crashing about... look forward to that happening. Being on an even keel.' BRIDIE

" 'First of all, I know it's rough at the moment, but when you get through it, it's better. And it's not just the absence of the menopause, but it can be better than it was before that as well. You know, it's something to look forward to. You know, don't fear it. It's something to look forward to. Life can be a lot better, can be a lot calmer. It can be, you know, there can be a point when you get to it and you think, wow, I didn't know it could actually be as good as this.' LILY

So be prepared and be reassured that menopause will end eventually (and we'll talk about what to expect, when it does, in Chapter 19). But what advice is there for coping with the process and symptoms of menopause, to help ease the transition through the menopausal journey? Our experts have insights relating to a number of different things that helped them navigate menopause, including advice about psychological factors (emotional and cognitive), coping strategies, finding information, exploring medical and non-medical options, dealing with doctors, and finding social support.

Be kind to yourself, keep a sense of humour and avoid rash decisions
The most common kind of advice our autistic experts gave us was about psychological factors. In particular, many people emphasized the importance of self-compassion and being kind to yourself, and gave examples of how to do this:

" 'If you're struggling, be kind to yourself. Simplify your commitments as far as possible. But kindness to yourself also means eating and exercising well.' SALLY

❝ 'Be kind to yourself. You are worth it. You are not your hormones.'
FLORENCE

❝ 'It's like, we often, you know, attend to the needs of teenagers and understand that they're going through a really difficult and profound change.
But we don't do that at the other end. We don't kind of go like, "oh, dear,
this woman's going through this enormous change of life". We just kind
of, "make certain to get on with it" while being mothers and carers and
partners and workers... we're not kind to women going through menopause. I think, you know, we need to really be kind to ourselves... buy all
the oils, buy all the linen clothes, you know, just give yourself what you
need during that time.' **ANNE**

❝ 'Really important to be kind to yourself because this is a really tough
period... don't beat yourself up because you're struggling. You know, it's
really a lot to cope with.' **DAISY**

❝ 'I would say it's really important [that] you're kind to yourself... don't compare yourself to a neurotypical person going through the menopause...
if you're thinking about all those other aspects like sensory needs, being
able to express yourself and sometimes not even being able to explain
your own feelings anyway, that's going to make it even harder for you.
Don't feel guilty about things you can't do for whatever reason, and don't
"compare and despair". Don't look at other people and think, "they seem
to be managing okay, I can't". I think it's just important to just recognize
that it's a journey and it's your own journey and you've just got to be kind
to yourself and help get through it really.' **ANN**

This is all sound advice. We know from research in non-autistic
people that self-compassion is very important for wellbeing during
menopause.[2] Emerging research in autistic people, too, suggests that
it can have 'life-changing' impacts on mental health.[3]

We know that for some readers, self-compassion will seem
impossible. It's a skill like any other – you might struggle to apply
it immediately, but it's something that you can develop proficiency
at. Tara had benefitted from meditative practices, which taught her
to appreciate even the tiniest 'upwards tilt' in her life:

" 'just those little decisions about can I get out of bed and go for a walk? And just really saying, well done, that was enough for today... I reflect back to friends [who are struggling] on the qualities they're demonstrating in just living their life rather than any big achievements.'

Exercising compassion for herself as well as others, Tara explained, was very much synonymous with feeling connected with others:

" 'When I'm sitting with whatever overwhelming experience I'm having, [I think] "okay, but if I'm having this overwhelming experience, there's so many human beings out there, there's no way I'm going to be alone in having this experience" – and actually acknowledge I'm working with this experience and communicating it, that in itself helps others because I know how much *I*'ve been helped by reading and listening to the experience of others. So there's a validation and connection through it because it can be so isolating thinking that you're totally on your own [with] your pain... being able to articulate it and live through this means that hopefully the next generation are going to have greater clarity and spaciousness... so there's that whole sort of mixture of spaciousness, compassion and connection, and it counteracts all of those sort of narratives that you can get into about "I'm so useless, I'm so alone", that can be so dangerous and drag you down further.'

Aside from self-compassion, other strategies or advice for psychological wellbeing were to 'take your sense of humour with you... you have to be able to laugh at what's happening' (Bassai Sho), and to avoid 'ridiculously rash decisions, [like] don't pack a suitcase and tell your husband to f*** off, then run away and join the circus. Put it off. Tell yourself "next year"' (The Cat).

Find coping skills that work for you
Just as our experts had very different experiences of menopause, they also told us about different approaches to coping with its symptoms. Part of being kind to yourself, in Anne's words, is 'giving yourself what you need', even if it might take some time to figure that out.

Lily had made great use of the gym, which helped her 'calm

things down a little bit'. Daisy used cold baths to combat brain fog, having procured a tub for her garden: 'It's horrible getting in, it's horrible getting out... but you feel so good after it. Tingling. The skin feels fresh... it's really something quite magical.' Alice had found ways of soothing herself when her emotions were raging and her mind was racing at night. She would play word games finding rhymes for simple words: 'I would go through each letter of the alphabet and think, can I make a word which rhymes with "take" and begins with this letter of the alphabet? The higher the score, the better.'

A number of our experts reflected that withdrawing from social encounters or potentially upsetting or stressful situations was a very important coping skill during menopause. It's not always easy to do this, or to give yourself permission to do it, but there's an increasing body of evidence showing that for autistic people, alone time is exceptionally important for 'regulating, recovering and recharging', so they can be 'ready to reconnect with others'.[4] Participants interviewed by Neville and colleagues, many of whom were autistic women in their 40s–50s, talked about the relief of escaping into cosy, safe spaces, controlled for sensory comfort, where they could immerse themselves in fiction or transcend into a focused flow state with their interests. For others in this study, making music, gaming, writing, gardening, photography, researching or learning something new were other ways of reaching a calming state of immersion. We now know that engaging in deep interests or passions is extremely important for wellbeing in autistic people.[5] As Ann advised, 'if you need more decompression time, take it'.

You heard our experts speak in Chapter 14 about developing paper or digital systems for remembering and organizing things (page 148). Janet advised autistic people going through menopause to:

> '... start writing, writing everything down. Download one of the checklists that you can get about menopause symptoms because that can, all of a sudden you can go, "oh, that's normal, that's normal, that's normal" because you don't, your brain isn't just going off... I think the main thing is just – write. Writing everything down where you can see, you can keep track of things, you can learn patterns.'

Learn as much as you can

Janet's suggestion taps into another vital coping strategy for many autistic people: many love to learn, explore and understand topics deeply and intricately, and may use this as a means of coping with uncertainty when they can't depend on professional help.[6] Our experts all highlighted the importance of understanding menopause, with some offering practical tools for finding information through relevant sources, though they noted that not all information will be relevant to everyone. For neurodivergent readers, information about neurodivergent experiences may be particularly helpful.

> 'I'd say educate yourself as much as possible. Look up several trusted sources, but remember menopausal experiences are as unique to you as your autism is, so not everything will apply to you... Don't assign any and every new symptom to your menopause – check out other possible causes.' SALLY

> 'Learn about it. Talk about it to people who will talk about it. Read about it. Just educate yourself.' BASSAI SHO

> 'Find out the information that you can, take as much time for yourself as you are able to, because I know it's not always possible... Don't panic... all of the changes are hard, but there are ways to ease in to this if you're kind to yourself. I think it's when things change or when strange and unusual things are happening in your body, it's very easy to just panic... Educate yourself and look after yourself. [There] is not really a lot else you can do. It's more of a "you're on the bus, you can't get off". You've just got to carry on until you get to the end of that journey.' SUZI

> 'I send people to the Davina McCall book and also the TV programmes. I found them very useful, both programmes that she did and also the My Menopause Centre [for details see the resources section at the end of the book]. I direct all my friends to that because they gave all this free information and the webinars and the newsletters and even the self-assessment checklist. It's all free... it really built my knowledge.' DAISY

We've also included some sources of further information at the end of this book.

Consider medical options...

There are mixed views about taking medication, particularly hormone replacement therapy (HRT), to help with the symptoms of menopause.[7] While consensus among experts is that the benefits ultimately outweigh potential costs for most people,[8] little is known about the efficacy and effects of HRT in minority groups, including neurodivergent people. Despite this, several of our autistic experts mentioned very positive experiences of HRT, while acknowledging the fear that autistic people might feel in trying new medication:

> 'The first lot of HRT I had gave me a lot of side effects and was unpleasant, but they swapped it around a couple of times and now I'm on something that actually does really help me. So, I would say don't discount HRT because it has been really useful for me, because if I could lessen some of the bodily symptoms, that helps with everything else.' SUZI

> 'Don't be frightened of it. It can really help and you can always try it. Come off it if you don't like it, but don't be frightened of that because, you know, it's quality of life. It's really made a big difference to me and I'll stay on it for as long as I can.' DAISY

> '... probably autistics more than many would be kind of worried about new things. One of the forums I'm on, a lot of people are really scared of HRT. And it's like, we do take a lot of things into our bodies. We do a lot of things that affect our bodies with our diet, etc.... But a lot of people, I think, are scared of HRT, again, partly because of historical and current studies. But... you can try it, and if it doesn't do something for you, you can tweak it. You can try different variations and actually... if you can see that through to thinking, "OK, it might not help immediately, but actually, over a process and time, if I put my faith in this and I actually am observant and see, okay, does it make a difference? Does it affect this? Does it help this, does it not?"... I don't think everything has been solved by HRT, but a lot of the major things have been helped. Definitely. So to kind of, to not be scared of that, not be scared of maybe trying, and trying a few things. I think that's important, too. Yeah, to be open.' KATIE

In qualitative work on autistic menopause, we and other researchers have spoken to autistic people who found HRT very helpful, as well as some who said that HRT was not for them.[9] Everyone has the right to choose. It's worth bearing in mind that although HRT can be taken at any point during the menopausal transition, many doctors believe that for HRT to be most beneficial, it is advisable to begin treatment sooner rather than later once menopausal symptoms begin.[10] You might remember, from earlier in this book, that Claire found her emotions heightened when she took HRT. She recognized that she had started taking it quite late, and expressed that things might have been better for her now if she had taken it sooner, advising that:

" 'Take the HRT as soon as possible and for as long as possible. Seek medical advice. I think that particularly female doctors now are a lot more knowledgeable about the menopause. And it is just a normal thing that every woman will go through it. It's just life, isn't it? So, yes, seek, seek medical advice. Take the drugs. That's good.'

... and be prepared to stand up for yourself in healthcare encounters

Several of our experts recognized the importance of medical support, but also the challenges that come with that. We know that unfortunately, autistic people often find themselves speaking a slightly different language to that of their doctors, making communication challenging.[11] On top of generally poor understanding of autism, there might be additional potential for difficulties at menopause,[12] given that doctors don't always agree with the best ways to manage symptoms.[13] As such, Florence wisely said: 'Don't be afraid to ask for help, but be prepared to have to stand up for yourself.' Asked what she wanted autistic people to know, Alice said:

" '... that doctors aren't always right... if you face resistance from your GP or if they try to just kind of fob you off, then you know, you don't have to accept that. Because I know for me... because I hate conflict, I hate fighting... so I just accepted what my GP said to me and in the end I just went private because I couldn't face the thought of trying to battle with my GP and persuade them to give me HRT. But, you know, there's tons of research on your side and there are also, you know, guidelines are changing for the NHS anyway that there are, there are guidelines out there by NICE [National Institute for

Health and Care Excellence] and that there are a lot of moves to make HRT more available and easy to get on the NHS. It isn't bad for you, it doesn't have to be bad for you and sometimes you have to be a little bit stubborn and bloody minded to get somebody to pay attention.'

Daisy also emphasized the importance of finding a supportive doctor and preparing yourself to ask for another doctor if necessary. In relation to healthcare generally, autistic people are often advised to write down what they want to say in advance or take an advocate with them.[14] Katie found this extremely helpful: 'I couldn't, couldn't express. I just couldn't. And my husband was fab... he had to just say, "No, she can't do this. She needs this. She needs this."'

Consider alternative treatment and supports

While some of our experts spoke about private medical care they'd benefitted from, others mentioned alternative treatments and therapies they had found helpful while navigating menopause and midlife:

66 '[I've got] a lovely autistic counsellor. We've done lots of work to try to really pull these things apart, and being able to put my experiences in the context of other autistic women. A lot of the stuff that was so scary beforehand, now I can recognize it and I have a lot more self-compassion about it and I've got strategies that are more appropriate.' TARA

66 'Luckily I'd been [seeing] a medicinal herbalist for many years... fortunately I had his support throughout, which I think saved me a little bit... I saw my herbalist, I went back and had some counselling, and I used to go and see my osteopath twice a month and just, you know, just realign everything, help with sleep...' ANNE

66 'I wish I'd known about acupuncture... it was a revelation for me... really helps me in lots of different ways, in my bone issues and my emotions.' DAISY

In the course of our research with autistic people, they've mentioned a range of other professionals, from professional organizers ('I learnt a life-changing amount of stuff'[15]) to naturopaths and complementary medicine.[16] We've noticed that the kinds of support most valued by autistic people are autism- and trauma-informed, and holistic, taking into account the full richness and complexity of the person's circumstances and health needs, being sensitive to what's said and unsaid.

Find social support... and your tribe

Finding social support was another area that all of our autistic experts highlighted as important in navigating menopause. Their advice included putting various types of support in place before things got really difficult; recognizing the need and giving oneself permission to ask for help; finding people to support you; and 'just to lean into any support available' (Anne).

❝ 'Working out how to put supports in place, and really trusting if things are starting to feel difficult. Try to work out options for supporting yourself and your family while you've still got the resources and the resilience to put in place new things. We've got a culture that's so much like, "everybody needs to be 100% busy or they are not valid members of society", but actually being 70% or less busy with 30% capacity to deal with, with a bit of creativity and a bit of spaciousness, particularly if you're autistic because of... a need to have more space around... Try to keep yourself below 70% capacity. And as soon as you start getting above that sort of 70% capacity, use that ability to put in place new things to take you below 70% so you don't have to get into the really desperate... Yeah, you got to put on your oxygen mask first, otherwise you're no help to anybody else.' TARA

❝ 'Find somebody to talk to who understands. The most important thing, I think, you know, is just somebody to walk with you.' LILY

❝ 'Find kind friends who can listen, particularly those that have gone through the menopause – they'll understand, you know, some of them will be really useful to you in terms of support.' DAISY

❝ 'It is okay to tell people, it's okay to talk about it and it's okay to ask for special treatment and consideration and help.' ALICE

❝ 'I think also trying to find someone who you can confide in and be honest with, because when you start to feel like you're just going... if you feel like you're going mad, you've got someone there... Yeah, just, just talk to someone. Because I think historically, for women going through the menopause, it can be extremely lonely anyway; for people who are already quite content to be quite isolated, I think it makes it worse.' JANET

❝ 'And I would say make sure you've got somebody like an ally or friend or family or a buddy that you can talk to because that does help. And share, share it. You know, don't hold it all in, you know, share with your friends, your family, your colleague, get somebody on your side to help you think as well.' ANN

Among sources of social support during menopause, autistic people express that the autistic community, naturally, has a special place.[17] Studies have shown that autistic-to-autistic communication is often experienced as more fluid, comfortable and enjoyable, and that autistic people find 'a certain magic' in the company of other autistic people.[18] We remember a participant who, when asked what autistic people need at menopause, said: 'Give them other autistic people who have been through the menopause. That's all.'[19] Another participant from the same study reflected on how helpful it was to hear from others who had struggled and 'walked the path back from Mad Land'.[20] Similarly, Bridie said she struggled with the kinds of 'empty platitudes' that are sometimes offered, and implied that it was more helpful to be around people who acknowledge the reality and magnitude of the difficulties while helping you feel that you are not alone.

Not all autistic people have friends they can meet in real life, but there are online spaces where autistic menopausal people can connect for this kind of support. Reflecting on the benefits of one online forum, Katie said that it could help a person see: 'It's not you going mad. There is a community of people and they may well have felt the same, similar, gone through the same as you. Also, it's not further evidence that you're broken. You're not. It's horrible, but it will pass.'

We hope that these messages from our experts will help autistic readers feel they are not alone, and that they can get through this time of life which can feel full of change and challenge. Look out for the bright sky after the turbulence, as Lily, Anne and Bridie said. On this note, we'll go on to consider the silver linings that our experts found at menopause.

Chapter 18

Positives of menopause...?!

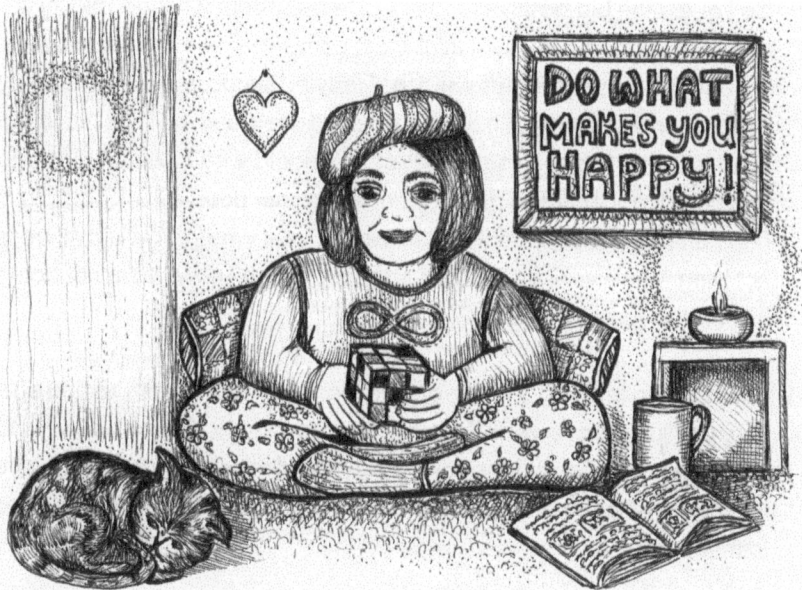

You might have read this chapter's title with some incredulity! Given the challenges we've discussed so far, some of you might be tempted to tell us to... flutter off. However, there were at least five key areas where our experts felt very definite positives around the experience of menopause and its symptoms, much like the 'silver linings' we identified in some of our earlier work.[1] If you'll remember back to Chapter 4 and the concept of menopause mindsets (page 45), having more positive thoughts and feelings about menopause (or less negative ones) may help people navigate the transition more smoothly.[2] As such, without wanting to dismiss or minimize the difficulties, we are keen to recognize the positives where they occur. Here are the positives our experts associated with their menopause experiences.

Caring less (but in a good way...)

Many of our autistic experts told us one of the positives of menopause was that they started to care less about what others thought of them and became less afraid of social judgement, and this particularly linked to their autism:

> 'So I guess the big positive for me: I care less about what people think... and I can be more me. And I think that's come from both the menopause, but also the autistic diagnosis and the lifestyle, I suppose... but more being able to confidently say, "I have autism and I see it and it affects me in this way" and, you know, also support other people who have autistic traits. So, yeah, [I] don't care so much about what other people think. You know, I do communicate differently to you, but it's not wrong. You know, we're not lying. We're very straightforward people. You know, we're not doing it to hurt anyone.' DAISY

> 'I think giving fewer f***s is one of them. Just, just not... I mean, as you age, you, you just give fewer f***s about stuff. You know, if someone says to me, Spike, you haven't done your hair, I just, I don't care. I just kind of care less about what other people think... So that's a positive when it comes to menopause.' SPIKE

You might remember from Chapter 15 (pages 156–158) that thankfully, along with their ability to mask, our experts' willingness to mask decreased. From stimming in public, wearing brighter clothes, talking about their interests, to dancing in the supermarket, our experts found that they were expressing their authentic selves more. In addition to the mask of neurotypicality, autistic people in our studies have reported feeling that menopause lifted the weight of societal pressures towards femininity, beauty and desirability.[3] One of our participants put it beautifully:

> 'Does it in fact drop away that layer of "I must prove myself, I must have this sparkling CV, I must be this beautiful woman?" Is the menopause a

moment when a woman is actually free to be herself? I don't know, but it has been for me.'[4]

A slowing down and acceptance of life and emotions

Something described as positive by many of our autistic experts was a sense of slowing down, feeling more accepting of life and their emotions. Through this, our experts described letting go and asserting their emotions in ways they felt were more healthy and authentic:

66 '... the positive has been slowing down and getting more of a life-work/ work-life balance. Doing classic things like gardening, you know? And I suppose another positive has been I've been a bit more reflective on life. But that's a tricky one because sometimes you can get caught up in, grieving the life that you probably won't have any more. I suppose maybe, maybe some of my words of wisdom to other people going through this is... your youth is now gone. Kind of just accept ageing, because I think that's one of the tough things about menopause is that, you know, that you're losing... you're kind of losing that life that you had. But there's a, there's a different life to be had now, a life where you can kind of hopefully slow down for other people's circumstances. Hopefully you can slow down, take stock and really identify what brings you joy and focus on that.' SPIKE

Both Suzi and Claire found themselves more able to express disagreement with other people. Suzi explained that whereas formerly, she would 'just go along' with 'something that was maybe a bit sexist or rude', 'now I just won't at all. I won't entertain any of that. I just tell [them], no, that's not the way it's going to be.' Similarly, Claire explained, that part of being 'more emotional' was her unwillingness to 'just soak up' things she disagreed with. Now, if someone snapped at her,

66 'I snap back... is it just because I'm not willing to put up with this crap any more? Put up with it for all my life. I'm not doing that any more. So... I'm more dysregulated, but maybe it's because I'm allowing myself to be dysregulated, whereas before I was possibly very controlled. And maybe one of the things I thought about being a healthy person was about controlling

your emotions and not allowing them to take over. Whereas now I'm kind of like, "let it all out. Just let it all out". Yeah, certainly that is a positive.'

Interestingly, this sense of slowing down and accepting your life is a feature of ageing,[5] and it's something that appears in the very few studies out there on ageing as an autistic person.[6] These studies suggest that some autistic people feel less social pressure, greater autonomy, and a sense of contentment, self-acceptance and self-compassion in later life, being more present-focused than worried about the future, a sense that life is good now.[7]

For some of our experts, this slowing down caused them to reflect on their identity and led to feelings of empowerment across many different areas of their life. They discovered a survivalist mentality, since having coped with the changes enforced on them by menopause, they felt empowered to make other positive changes in their life:

> '[Menopause] kind of enabled/forced me to confront my identity. And I think that's incredibly empowering... it has explained so much. Not just now, but in retrospect, it's like, OK, "this is why I did feel like that". And it's probably forced me to reach out to a community, both [an] autistic community and menopausal community, which perhaps wouldn't have been my natural kind of instinct. But sometimes you need to... something makes you ultimately go, "okay, actually there is this stuff out there, there's people out there", and you can dip in and out, put your toe in the water a little bit in terms of that community. Yeah, it has made that happen. And I think having had to address physical/emotional change has actually emboldened me to seek new directions in my job, but also more widely. I'm somebody who's got faith, a very strong faith. And... you kind of go, okay, well, I've lived through the last couple of years and I haven't died yet. I haven't wanted this change, but I can cope with some of this change. Maybe, actually, I can make some more positive changes myself. I can find something which is better. Now I very strongly feel that... so you have to find positives and you have to find, okay, what's my way through this? This will end, something better will come of it. It has to.' KATIE

These kinds of sentiment are things we've seen in participants in our studies. One, despite the mental health struggles of menopause, described it as a 'springboard for me to do amazing things';[8] another described it as 'a time of remaking my identity... that let the light of autism out after decades of squishing it deep down'.[9]

Pruning and refining your relationships

As you might remember from Chapter 15 (page 152–153), many of our experts were much more selective in their socializing, as a consequence of menopause. Some, who had previously been people-pleasers, diplomats and nurturers, described a positive of menopause in the pruning of relationships that were no longer serving them. This allowed them to save their resources and focus on their own coping and self-care. When you think back to the research we spoke about in Chapter 5 (page 58), that menopausal women who self-silenced in their relationships showed more signs of health problems,[10] then this new boldness feels like a wonderful development! We've heard these kinds of feelings and experiences expressed again and again by research participants, who were no longer prepared to accept ill-treatment:[11]

> 'I find there is a place for me in this world – it's the place/space I give myself to be me. No one who disagrees will be listened to.'[12]

> 'I put up with less crap from so called friends and some family, and eventually I got rid of some of those relationships. Life was too short to waste it on people who didn't really care, weren't actually very pleasant or who were just using me for whatever reasons.'[13]

Along with the pruning of negative relationships, several of our experts developed new relationships that served them, or found existing relationships strengthened or 'galvanized', in Anne's words (page 159). For some, menopause appeared to give them a connecting point from which to relate to others:

> 'In the same way that when you are experiencing anything, you can sort of find people that you didn't know were there or that you needed... in the same way, I found, you know, mostly just online, and found people who are sympathetic... And you just find a different sort of relationship with people,

some of them are strangers, some of them are perhaps people that you just... didn't know about. And in a way it's quite nice and to some extent it has slightly improved my relationship with other women, because I was bullied a lot at school by other groups of girls... because I've never quite fitted in... this area, which felt a bit difficult for me, you know, interacting with other women... But yeah, it's enabled me to sort of heal that part of myself, if that makes sense... I've got a different kind of closeness with my father, which I've never, ever had before.' JANET

66 'Closeness with other middle-aged women. Being able to share your experiences and stuff has brought me and other friends closer, and even the male friends actually, who've been very kind and listened.' DAISY

66 'Having two daughters, I was able to go through the whole menstrual cycle with them, kind of? Not a bonding experience, but... now with the menopause. I get to go through growing a moustache and beard with my son. So yeah, it's really positive.' BASSAI SHO

For some of our autistic experts, they developed greater empathy for others going through menopause and felt better able to reach out and help them:

66 'I think the positive is... that I have a much better understanding... I like to think that I can really feel more support and empathy for anybody who is going through it or who is perimenopausal, whereas before I might have sort of gone, "Oh yeah, you know, that's not very nice, is it?" and not really thought much more about that. Whereas now I think I would really be able to take time and understanding how that is impacting that that person... And also, you know, being able to share, you know, "this was helpful", "this wasn't that helpful", you know... I think now that I'm in it myself, I feel like I can maybe help other people who are going through or entering it. So that's a positive.' ANN

Freedom from periods

One physical positive of going through menopause, mentioned frequently by our experts and participants in research studies, is being free from periods and all they entail.[14] Those going through

POSITIVES OF MENOPAUSE...?!

perimenopause were encouraged by the prospect of periods ending, particularly given the difficulties that autistic people report around menstruation.[15] In Bridie's words, periods ending meant an 'even keel' 'without hormones crashing about', and an end to the cycle of:

> 'one week of a month where you might just about feel okay and the other times you're either pre-period or post period... either coming from a place of huge hormonal influx into your system and then you have your period, which is ghastly, then you've got the post-period week and a bit, and then you've got like five days of going, "Oh, thank god, just be me, just be normal. Just be me." Then it all starts again'.

Others shared this feeling:

> 'I love the fact that there's no more periods. Because with the heavy periods, you are just so done with it... Yeah, I find it very positive, very freeing. I can finally wear white.' BASSAI SHO

> '... when my periods actually go away. I'm looking forward to that day so that will be a positive thing, because actually having difficult periods every month is probably difficult for autistic people anyway because your body just is in uproar all of a sudden and you're like, "Oh, I'm here again and everything's difficult." So not having periods will be a positive, I think.' SUZI

Some autistic people we've spoken to, who really suffered with their periods, felt like menopause 'was rediscovering a body that had no periods, that I hadn't encountered since I was 12... all of the kind of years between, when I was like up and down, up and down emotionally and in bed with pain and bleeding and anaemic, I think, "yeah it was a phase, it was a very long phase, but this feels more like the real me"'.[16] Notably, those going through menopause who do not identify as women or who feel uncomfortable with that identity are likewise probably going to experience the cessation of periods as a relief, an end to the 'gender tug' or 'battle that's going on' (Lily).

191

A learning process of self-discovery and growth

As you saw in Chapter 9, some of our experts, and our research participants, expressed a sense of gratitude that menopause had led to the realization of their autism, albeit via a rocky road of turbulence. One of our participants, reflecting on the self-acceptance and self-compassion that came with this realization, said: 'I feel as if I've been on a journey, um, which contained many different facets and has resulted in me being brave enough to be me.'[17] Travelling this road meant that some participants from that study were now able to be 'more selfish and more controlled', or 'more aware of needing those days where I'm just binge-watching box sets... having massive downtime, and not feeling guilty for it... thinking, "you know what, this is actually what you need", and just embrace it'.[18] Across several of our studies, and as expressed by some of our experts, better self-understanding had led to the development of greater resilience, new coping skills, and greater ability to protect themselves and give themselves what they needed.[19]

Along with the benefits of realizing a neurodivergent identity, some of our autistic experts also pointed to the positive benefit of menopause also enabling them to understand more about other ongoing health conditions. Daisy described her growing understanding of the complex and intersecting relationships between neurodivergence, physical health issues and menopause as 'like unwrapping an onion, finding a piece of info that leads to another to another until we have the whole picture'. Although private medical investigations had been extremely expensive, she did not regret having found out about these things, and said one positive of menopause was:

❝ 'I guess because I was so bad, with so many different health issues, it allowed me to get to the bottom of all my health issues. Before, I had found coping mechanisms for most of my issues for most of my life... menopause changed that, as everything blew up, so it wasn't possible to just continue with the status quo. And now I feel that I have a really good picture of why I've had so many different problems in my life... yeah, so I guess it's allowed me to understand better.... [Getting these other diagnoses] felt like having bags of cement removed from my shoulders. Just knowing the reasons of some of the symptoms was so important and freeing.'

There were other positives mentioned by our experts, although less consistently. Some, for example, found relief in the cessation of sex, while others expressed sadness in the loss of desire. We've also heard from autistic people who've enjoyed a second flush of youth in heightened sexuality and libido during and after menopause.[20]

Since the challenges of menopause understandably receive the most air-time, we feel it's important to know that, just as our experts said, there is a way through, and it's not all bad. Thinking back to menopause as the crossroads we spoke about in Chapter 5, we've heard from some autistic people who, despite struggling with self-harm and suicide during menopause, traversed into a better life afterwards:

66 'I'm just starting to blossom now. I'm 50 this year and I'm taking off now so it's great!... I mean there's still a lot to do but you know, umm, I just want people to know that the menopause is not the end of your life.'[21]

This feels like a good time to talk about life postmenopause, the focus of our next chapter.

Chapter 19

Life on the other side of menopause

Postmenopausal experiences

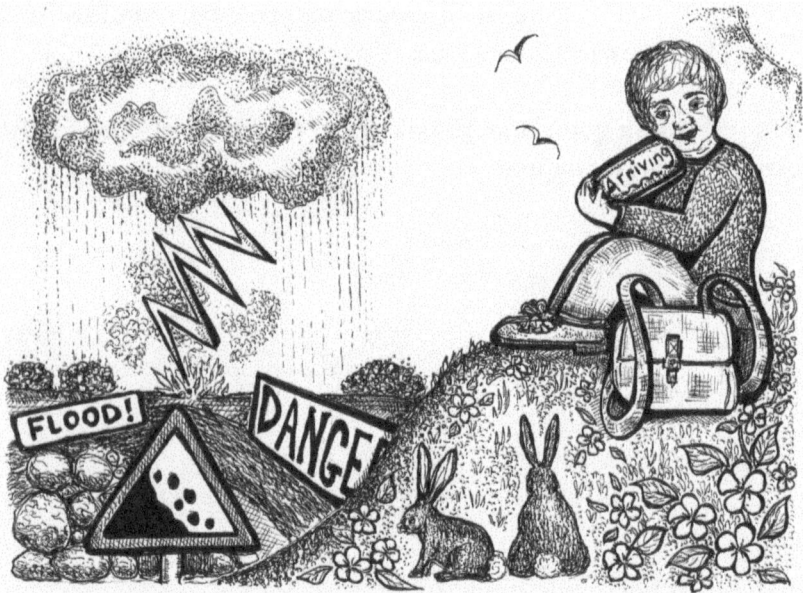

We asked those of our experts who were postmenopausal to describe how they felt on the other side of menopause. While the topic of menopause has increasingly enjoyed media visibility and academic attention in the past few years, there is relatively little information and support focused on life on the other side of menopausal symptoms, where we talk of people being postmenopausal. Claire pointed out:

❝ '... what I struggle with now and what frustrates me a little is that the focus, a lot of the focus now is on the menopause, on that transition. No one's really talking about after and I, in my head, I kind of thought... I know it's a transition. I know it's a change. But in my head, I thought I'd go back to how things were before.'

As you can imagine and as Claire's quote shows, holding these kinds of mistaken beliefs could lead to a lot of frustration, confusion and disappointment when menopause ends. It's extremely easy to see why Claire thought that things would go back to her old normal. The hormonal upheaval of menopause is often viewed by others (family, friends, medical professionals/healthcare providers) as over or having finished once people reach the postmenopausal stage.

If you think back to the STRAW+10[1] stages of menopause that we mentioned at the start of this book (pages 26–27), you might remember that there are actually several stages of postmenopause. The 'early' stages of postmenopause are approximately the first 4–5 years after your last period, during which that increasingly disjointed dance between the hormones produced in the brain and those produced in the ovaries is going on. The brain is still pumping out follice stimulating hormone (FSH) but the ovaries can't respond and estrogen continues to decrease. As late postmenopause is reached, high FSH and low estrogen stabilize and largely remain in this state of play for the rest of the lifespan.

You probably gathered from this that it's common for the smorgasbord of menopausal symptoms (vasomotor symptoms, psychological changes to emotion and cognition, sleep problems and urogenital symptoms) to continue at least through early postmenopause, where vasomotor symptoms may actually be most likely,[2] although symptoms as a whole might not be as intense and bothersome as in perimenopause.[3] Though some of these symptoms cease altogether in late menopause, some researchers suggest that people continue to sleep less[4] and experience continued urogenital symptoms as they age.[5]

This is what research tells us about broad populations but not specifically neurodivergent ones. The uncertainty of postmenopause may be particularly difficult for autistic people, whose world may have changed dramatically, who have no certainty about the road ahead, and who might now be newly aware of their autism following a diagnosis, alongside other health conditions. The invisibility of autistic elders leaves some people worried about the ageing process, without any role models to 'show me that getting older isn't something to be frightened of'.[6]

Our experts generously shared their experiences to shine a light on this life stage. We weren't able to identify which stage of postmenopause they were in (which might explain something of the variety of experiences), but what we perceived was a shift from the rollercoaster experienced during the height of menopause to the swings and roundabouts of the later postmenopause as symptoms began to decline and settle into a 'new normal'. What was apparent were the mixed views and experiences, with individuals often reporting both positive and negative aspects.

Making sense of life postmenopause

Our experts, like other autistic people, hadn't benefitted from a roadmap through perimenopause and into postmenopause. Some described still trying to figure things out and make sense of their life postmenopause, often unable to discern which experiences were related to menopause and which to midlife circumstances and demands, as Tara explained:

" '[I] still feel as if I'm picking up the pieces. And... have not got a stable situation at all. And I can talk a little bit about the different elements of that [work, pension, elderly parents, supporting teenage children]... the expectation of being able to be consistent, to manage other people's expectations... it just made me really sick. So there's trauma, there's autistic burnout, there's late diagnosis. How much of that is menopause? I don't know... So at the moment, life's feeling fairly tough... dry humour and kindness are sort of, just the ways of getting through it all, and just going, "okay, how do I prioritize things that feel meaningful and are supportive, and how do I try and make those sensible choices about not having the extra glass of wine or the ice cream?" And working out, having enough energy to find places to build in the additional support... so yes, as ever, can't say what is menopause and not menopause related.'

Some readers might ask if it matters whether these feelings and experiences are related to menopause, ageing or autism diagnosis: do you really need to know the cause? The answer, for many autistic people, is very simply 'yes'. Linking back to that drive for certainty and predictability, autistic people typically want to understand, with great clarity and precision, what is happening to them and why. Being unable to understand has serious mental health impacts, as Claire explains:

> 'This is why I think coming out of the menopause, this is why I really struggled with my mental health, because now I find it really hard to unpick what's the menopause, what's ADHD, what's autism, what's attachment, what's just me? – because of the person I am, I want to understand myself. I want to know, I want the answers, or maybe the answers aren't out there... so, I think that undermined my sense of self a little bit.'

Positives at postmenopause: discovering support, enjoying calmer waters

Our experts mentioned several unexpected benefits of postmenopausal life. First, some reported receiving enormous postmenopause support and kindness, particularly from the autistic and neurodivergent community that they had discovered during menopause:

> '... my tribe ... suddenly I found... a huge bunch of menopausal and postmenopausal neurodivergent women. It has been very fun.' SALLY

> 'the number of other women I talk to... thinking they're going mad... [In] the autism world... there's enormous kindness... when you meet certain people because it's like, "This is all crap. The support systems are all crap. The prospects don't look great. OK, let's just laugh and move on"... [Refers to a poem]... Getting through the despair and I'm finding some kindness.' TARA

Some of our experts also reported feeling better in themselves – the word 'calm' came up several times, from Lily, Sally and Anne, while Bridie expressed her relief at being on an 'even keel' after the end of periods, as you saw in the previous chapter. Sally described menopause as being 'stormy, [then] you get into calm waters and it's nice', describing a stark contrast with the earlier, most symptomatic stages of menopause: 'There's a whole beautiful "new you" waiting at the other side, when you get through it. I mean, that is postmenopause, that is. Menopause itself, I wouldn't wish it on my worst enemy.'

Some of our experts even felt better than they'd felt before menopause, as Anne described, and which strikes a chord with what we previously mentioned about social expectations placed on women (e.g. pages 48 and 184):

66 'It's not like this any more [indicates the up and down rollercoaster], it's kind of, you know [indicates a flat line]. This might be really abstract, but I feel like when I was a child... [having described being very "self-assured" and relatively unaffected by bullying and othering]. But when puberty started, that all changed. I really started to feel very self-conscious about myself and being weird... I really started to be like really acutely aware of it for the first time. And that was pervasive, right through most of my adult female life, this feeling of external scrutiny, of "that's not what women do. That's not how women act. That's not how women look. That's not how women sound. That's not what women say. That's not what women do." And I really felt quite oppressed by that for a long time. And all the monkey business... worrying about things like being attractive and the sexuality stuff... I just feel free of it, I feel like I did when I was a child. I feel liberated. Where I'm kind of the person that I was meant to be before people started and wrecked everything, the person that maybe I should have been, because I don't feel any of that othering and I don't feel any of that oppressive scrutiny.'

We've heard feelings of freedom and liberation like this before, from the quotes you heard in the previous chapter from our research participants.[7] Some, like Anne, felt more like themselves than they had before the rollercoaster of hormones began at puberty. One participant told us her 'quality of life [was] much better' (than during menopause), and she'd been able to pick up, again, the coping skills that had been derailed by cognitive dysfunction. She said: 'In some ways I'm doing better now than I ever have really, I think I'm more comfortable in my own skin now than I ever was.'[8]

Disadvantages and disappointment

For some, though, this calmness co-existed with disadvantages and disappointment at the continuation of menopausal symptoms, as Sally expressed: '[Life is] calmer, but since having all estrogen stripped from my body, I miss feeling desire.'

As you saw earlier, some of our experts found the continuation of symptoms, and change in their functioning, an unpleasant, unexpected surprise, having thought they'd 'be normal again' (Claire). Autistic people certainly won't be alone in this unpleasant surprise, given poor menopause education broadly, and the invisibility of the postmenopause stage. We've spoken to other autistic people who were disappointed to not return to their premenopause state. One, having explained that hot flushes, insomnia, aches and pains, heightened sensory sensitivities and cognitive dysfunction had all diminished or stopped, said:

> 'I would say that I'm improving slowly... but I don't know whether I will ever get back to what I used to be able to do, in terms of output and in terms of productivity, in terms of concentration. I've got a lot of work-arounds that I have to use, and a lot of supplements and a lot of other things that I have to do these days to be able to sustain it... I'm left being a very, very tired person all the time... It takes so much stuff to keep me functioning... okay.'[9]

So, swings and roundabouts in postmenopause? Well, it certainly did sound like our experts experienced postmenopause as a relief from the worst of the menopausal symptom rollercoaster, but some still yearned for their previous state or experienced continuing symptoms. Unfortunately, it's very hard to get that clear roadmap, as the experiences of our experts undoubtedly were influenced by their postmenopausal stage (and relatedly, symptom levels), their health and treatment received during perimenopause, and by other events and circumstances.

Claire said that it was very important for autistic people to be aware that symptoms don't stop completely, and one's state doesn't revert once they hit postmenopause. We strongly agree but hope that the consensus of getting off the rollercoaster, the improvements to life post periods and postmenopause, and indeed the positive experiences reported by some autistic people, will show readers that there is most definitely hope and perimenopause won't last forever!

Chapter 20

Advice for professionals supporting autistic people through menopause

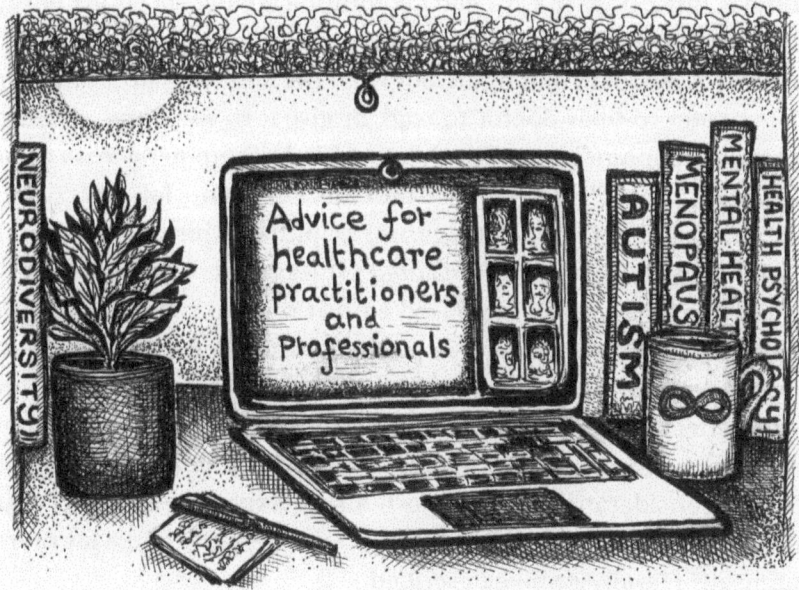

A consistent finding across our studies and those of other researchers is that autistic people often run into difficulties when seeking support, healthcare or otherwise, during menopause.[1] Many struggle through without support, due to professional disinterest, knowledge gaps or inaccessible services, and some were harmed by the responses they received. As such, we wanted to turn the tables and ask our autistic experts what they would like to tell professionals about menopause as experienced by autistic people. Healthcare professionals like general practitioners (GPs) in the UK (equivalent of a primary care physician in the USA) featured very prominently in their answers, as did the National Health Service and healthcare provision more generally. However, their responses are relevant to a much wider group of professionals who work with autistic people across different sectors.

This chapter is not only intended for healthcare providers and other professionals supporting autistic people through menopause. It will also empower autistic people to self-advocate, and assist those who support them to help advocate for them, in the very often challenging landscapes of health and social care. For example, in healthcare settings, autistic readers might, for instance, like to highlight those bits that apply to them (e.g. 'even though I'm saying "yes, everything is fine... it wasn't"'; 'I can't communicate my emotions or my symptoms effectively ... [the medical profession is] going to have to work with me to try and figure out what the heck they are') and give the chapter to their doctor to read, or give it to someone who can attend an appointment with them and help them get across what they want to say. You might also find the 'Key points for professionals' at the end of the book (page 218) helpful for this purpose, too.

What our autistic experts wanted professionals to know was very much focused around increased education and training, both in menopause and autism, and in particular the intersection between autism and menopause. They felt it was impossible to separate out which effects were due to menopause and which to autism, and that 'autistic menopause' was, in fact, a category in itself that needed greater consideration and support. All our experts recognized that autistic menopause 'can be experienced differently and a lot more intensely' (Tara). As Spike described:

❝ 'Autistic people going through the menopause might not be able to identify all the things that are classic symptoms. And we can't separate the autistic from the menopause as well. I think that's the big thing, autistic menopause is a thing in itself. It's not just being autistic and it's not just being menopausal. It's autistic menopause.'

Healthcare professionals need better education on menopause and health for women and people assigned female at birth

As we mentioned earlier, there's huge variation in professional knowledge and attitudes about menopause, even among doctors.[2] Our experts clearly experienced this in reality, and there was a strong sense that healthcare practitioners need to know more about menopause and women's health in general,[3] and the impact that menopause can have in order to provide better care. Among other comments, Daisy expressed:

> 'They need to know about the perimenopause and that it can start from the early 40s and for a few women before this. They need to be trained... half the population will go through this condition. And it's so devastating for people... I would want professionals to know that it can have a massive effect on people's lives. And something that struck me... the highest rate of suicide for females in age bracket is 45 to 50. And when you know about how little support there is for people with perimenopause and I know about like mine and my friends' experiences of how our lives have been turned upside down.'

Professionals need to update their knowledge on autism and neurodivergence in adults

Overwhelmingly, our autistic experts strongly emphasized the need for health professionals, as well as those across other professions, to be educated about and trained in autism and neurodivergence (particularly in people assigned female at birth), and the particular differences that autistic people may present with at menopause. As Sally put it, medical professionals need to understand 'what it means to be an autistic woman, as opposed to what they were taught in medical school in their one-hour lecture [on] autism'. This fits with what we know from research: healthcare professionals receive training focused on autistic children and are less knowledgeable and confident about working with autistic adults, particularly those assigned female at birth.[4]

Our experts found that they often ran up against misconceptions or knowledge gaps in the professionals who were meant to be helping them. For example:

❝ 'I've been in lots of different meetings or discussions where I've talked about alexithymia and they go, "I don't know what that is." And I go, well, you know, you work in mental health, you need to, you need to know about it. Because if you're doing questionnaires every week with someone and they're saying, "I don't understand, I don't know what to write for the answer," and you're getting frustrated... you're not delivering what you should be delivering in a way that somebody understands it, you haven't done your research. So there's no point you getting frustrated with your patient.' ANN

❝ 'I would just like health professionals to get some actual proper training in autism and specifically female autism... if people have a level of understanding of autistic women, they will automatically have more of an understanding of autistic women in the menopause. I've dealt with [GP, doctors at hospital, people at work, occupational health, people in my union]... None of them, not one single person has any training in autism... everybody that I've spoken to has thought it was a mental health condition. And I've had to explain. "No, it's not. It's a structural difference. It can cause mental health problems. It can cause all these other problems"... and I still get asked, "So what drugs are you taking?" And "is it likely to go away?"... even the people in the disability network don't think autism is a proper disability. And it actually does really affect everything in your life... somebody needs to force people who work in health and wellbeing to do this training because there are so many autistic people... women are being found like me, in later life... [without training] women who are autistic will never get what they need.' SUZI

Our experts also pointed out that training should specifically include cross-neurotype communication barriers between autistic and non-autistic people, as well as difficulties autistic people might experience in communicating or expressing their symptoms and how they feel during menopause. They spoke about this especially in the context of healthcare, as you'll see.

Healthcare professionals need to know about the intersection of autism and menopause, and must show greater understanding and empathy

Our experts made frequent mentions of healthcare encounters in the context of menopause, and subsequently called for more understanding, awareness and empathy for autistic people going through menopause, especially since, as Katie pointed out, some autistic people will be unable to self-advocate. This is what our experts wanted from healthcare practitioners:

" '... [to know that] there's a very high chance we're experiencing it differently to how textbook women experience menopause, and to just have a little bit more... understanding that we're not being difficult or neurotic. And when we do seek help, it's because we're coming from a place of not understanding more than arrogance or anything like that.' BASSAI SHO

" '... to understand, or for there to be a greater knowledge of women's specific health issues... because even for menopause, it is still a struggle to find the right person... And I feel like even if there was a better understanding of... [the] presentation of neurodivergent women and the varying aspects of menopause... Just to understand how strongly it can impact on your mental health... sometimes I just feel like I would just like them to consider something at all, if that makes sense.' JANET

" '... more awareness and more empathy. You actually need to care about your patients and treat them as human beings rather than numbers to tick off your list for your ten-minute appointment... if somebody said to me, "who's the least, who is that profession that you most distrust?" I would say doctors. Which is sad, really, isn't it? Because we used to say that doctors were like the most trustworthy, respected, highest.' DAISY

Unfortunately, across research studies, autistic people assigned female at birth particularly report feeling dismissed by health professionals.[5] Older autistic people have also reported feeling like their healthcare needs are regarded as less important,[6] so it's possible that our experts were experiencing being at the intersection of several disadvantaged identities, just like the participant we quoted on page 85, who queried whether poor treatment at work was 'because

I am a woman, an ageing woman, or an ageing autistic woman who has been treated for cancer.' Our experts asked of healthcare professionals:

" '... [to] not be dismissive [or] invalidating, and to understand that if you're autistic and you're menopausal, they need to see that together and not, "oh, over there is autism and over there is menopause"... professionals need to be mindful of understanding where that woman or person is coming from, from their autistic self as well. Instead of "wow, oh, you know, most women report this". Well, you're not most women... sometimes it's difficult to explain your feelings and your thoughts or what's happening with your body. You don't know why you think or feel like that. I think offering some validation, some reassurance, and don't be dismissive of somebody's autistic experience because within the professional world, there's almost a... "we, we don't mention the autistic bit, okay? Because everybody's equal and everybody's included"... it happens a lot in mental health and primary care, it's brushed aside like.' ANN

" '... to be aware that if you already struggle with emotional regulation... executive function... concentration and memory... all of that is going to be exacerbated by the menopause and there is going to be a complex interaction between [autism and menopause]. So don't assume that it's just more neurodivergence. It might be being exacerbated by hormonal fluctuations. So pay attention to that and be understanding about, for instance, how it can already be difficult for somebody newly [diagnosed] neurodivergent to communicate and particularly to communicate with professionals. And if they are also suffering with problems with memory, concentration and emotional dysregulation, that is going to make all of that even harder, really stressful and they're going to need some consideration. They don't want to be patronized, but they also don't want to be fobbed off... think about how hard it can be to get yourself to a medical or health professional in the first place. And if then they're not listening to you or they're just fobbing you off, that, that's actually incredibly stressful and distressing.' ALICE

Our experts emphasized that the autistic community are the greatest source for learning how to work appropriately with autistic people. Bridie said that speaking to those with lived experience is 'the only way that the medical profession is going to move on... from diagnosis to assessment to everything to do with autistic people, until they get that lived experience, talking to them, nothing will change, unfortunately.' Daisy agreed, saying:

" 'Listen to them... don't snap, speak down, fob off, be arrogant, basically don't assume that you know more than your patients. You know, the point is to work with them... use their knowledge and use your knowledge, particularly with rare diseases, but also with the menopause.'

Professionals need to listen to autistic people – and believe them

Indeed, what was stressed several times by our autistic advocates was the need to be believed. While this seems like a small and fundamental thing, autistic people across research studies have expressed that, in a menopause context and in relation to broader mental/ physical health, their distress was misunderstood and disregarded by professionals, often because they weren't conveying it in expected ways.[7] It is essential to listen to the words, even if they're not being said in a way you would normally associate with distress. Many of our experts felt they were not believed or taken seriously in healthcare situations, which undermined their ability to get help:

" 'I want professionals to believe us when we say how we feel. Be kind to us. Don't be dismissive or belittle how we are feeling, because we will remember that and it will live with us, sometimes for years. It may even affect our ability to seek medical help when we need to. We are experts in who we are.' FLORENCE

" '... you're treated as though you're just making things up and you're just an annoying middle-aged woman... [Having referred to suicide rates in the 40–50s age bracket] I want them to care about that... I want to say, women won't come to you... because it's very unpleasant to be fobbed off by a doctor, to not be listened to, to be made to feel your problems are not important. So if they come to you, then they really have a problem... it's not hysterical women... and autistic menopausal women wouldn't come to see you unless they really, really needed help.' DAISY

" 'Just because I can't communicate my emotions or my symptoms effectively doesn't mean they're not real. And [the medical profession is] going to have to work with me to try and figure out what the heck they are. You know, you're going to have to go through a list of things, "Is it this is it, is it this?" That might be tedious for you, but I'm sorry. I wish I could give you more, but I can't because I experience these symptoms and I can't articulate them. It doesn't mean I'm crazy, [or] attention seeking, [or] a hypochondriac, [or] hysterical, all of which have been thrown at me... you need to stop bringing your own prejudices and your own assumptions to the consultation because you're damaging your patient's physical and mental health by doing that.' LILY

Professionals need to offer additional support in medical settings

This difficult-to-disentangle enmeshment, between autism features and menopause symptoms, brought to light the training and education needs in healthcare providers. Our autistic experts were able to describe some clear additional support that would help with this in medical settings, principally time: time for greater discussion, explanation about medication and treatment, and communication support to get the information patients needed – much reminiscent of our research studies, where, for instance, participants explained, 'I need encouragement and support to be able to ask questions in a healthcare setting, and because I don't receive this, I often don't ask questions that I would like to'.[8] This is especially important when we remember that many autistic people will enter menopause with limited understanding of its nature and what it entails. Our experts also highlighted the need for better understanding and coordinated support for other ongoing, complex and intersecting health issues and above all, continual, proactive and preventative care. Here's what they said:

" 'In terms of... making it easy for autistic women to know what the options are and to support them, I'd imagine it's... about talking about the symptoms, looking at the different options, and then through a trial and error basis, working through them and seeing what helps. And it may be that because of the disproportionate potential impact on autistic women, they should get fast-tracked access and additional support... I wish that I'd had confidence that the GP could have said, "Right, you're coming up to menopause, your depression symptoms are increasing, you're struggling at work, you know, let's get you some sessions with a specialist, we'll look at what the options are"... And... the heterogeneity of the autistic population and the sensory sensitivities and the latest information... it would have been nice for my GP to know that.' TARA

" '... I need more time. I need to ask questions. I need to talk about/understand the details. Because unless I understand the details and/or triangulate to make sense, I won't believe them.' DAISY

" '... I didn't really understand what the purpose of HRT was [when it was first discussed]. I just thought that HRT was to minimize your menopausal symptoms. And I kind of thought, well, at some point I have to stop taking the HRT and those symptoms will come back and I'll have to go through it. So let's just get it over and done with... I didn't understand the role of estrogen in the brain and how it might benefit me... if I knew what I know now, I would have taken the HRT as early as possible and stayed on it for as long as possible because I possibly wouldn't be in the mess that I'm in now.' CLAIRE

The following comment reminds us that healthcare professionals need to be aware of the very significant likelihood that autistic people will present with complex co-occurring and possibly interrelated conditions, diagnosed and/or undiagnosed, which might be exacerbated by menopause (as we saw in Eunhee Kim's work on page 125):

" 'You know, we need specialist care because we've probably got more than likely physiological conditions that maybe we don't even know about... things like hypermobility syndrome, they're going to get significantly worse during menopause. We may not know. We may not know what the symptoms are, and we might need somebody to sit down and ask us specifically, "are you experiencing insomnia, are you experiencing brain fog?" [indicates realization] "Oh, it's that, that's what it is." You may need it spelt out... And I think you need regular appointments with somebody to ground you in that. Not just once where somebody goes, "do you want some HRT?" and you say, "no thanks," and they say, "right, see you then". You know, you may need a regular appointment with somebody where you go to the same person, where you go and you talk about how it's changed... there's this feeling of... women should just deal with this on their own somewhere, especially autistic women... it was very isolating. And just understanding how isolating it is, maybe for people who don't have those networks that you would expect... It's my belief that we need specialist gynaecological care right from the get-go, from young people starting their period... there's lots of things that maybe need to be thought about... autistic people going through menopause need ongoing specialist care.' ANNE

Professionals must reduce barriers to healthcare in autistic menopause

Our experts mentioned a number of additional barriers which made it difficult for them to access help, particularly from the NHS. Alice, like some of our other experts and research participants,[9] sought private medical care because accessing HRT 'from my GP was so complicated and difficult'. She said:

" 'The NHS is in a state of crisis, I get this, but trying to sort it out so that I could get it from the pharmacy was just so hard. [A friend] was told by her GP that hormonal prescriptions have to be renewed once a month, whereas her husband is on medication that he can renew every three months. And given how hard it is to get a prescription, to get it fulfilled by the pharmacy, to get the paperwork sorted out, to even get hold of a GP on the phone or via any other means, to be forced to do that once a month is just insane... hard for any woman who's going through menopause. But if you're also autistic, which makes communication, dealing with people, phone calls... a lot of that stuff is already hard. Like don't put more barriers in the way. It's just not fair, you know?'

Others pointed to the barriers created through what might now be common practice in healthcare, such as phone consultations, although some autistic people prefer these.[10] Katie described phone consultations as 'atrocious', because when she was asked how she was:

" 'I could just about say, "okay". And it wasn't, it wasn't okay... if I'd known

I was autistic, I might have said, "no" or I might have said, "no, I need to see somebody rather than speak to somebody over the phone", because then you can actually see that I'm not okay. Even though I'm saying, "yes, everything is fine", because it wasn't. But also that not everyone will be able to describe their emotions.'

Katie also highlighted that 'treatment as usual' may be inappropriate and inaccessible for autistic people. While CBT has an evidence base in reducing menopause symptoms,[11] we know that in the context of mental health conditions, CBT can be unhelpful for autistic people when delivered in an un-adapted form.[12] Presently, we simply don't know the best psychological support for neurodivergent people during menopause, but psychological interventions which do not understand or respect autistic culture may risk invalidating the experiences of this already marginalized group,[13] as Katie explained:

" 'I did CBT [cognitive behavioural therapy]... I actually insisted on the C-CBT [computerized/internet-delivered CBT], the online one, because I didn't want somebody, a therapist, to say, "actually, can you challenge your thoughts?" And I'd say, "no – because this is real". This is, this is what is real. This is not something which is, kind of... I'm used to thinking I'm wrong. And actually, I am being really honest and being really... when I'm telling you this is the case, this is the case. Please believe me. I think that, that one size will not fit all, I suppose, and that has to be taken into account. But again, that comes back to kind of would it help to know that you're autistic before you go through menopause? Yeah, yeah it would!'

Although our experts were asked about their advice for professionals, we recognize that many of these goals actually depend on action from higher legislative bodies to provide the training and resources needed. These inadequacies in public services have real and serious consequences. Though some of our experts were able to seek private healthcare and found this helpful, some mentioned the severe financial repercussions of this necessity. For many, this pathway will not be an option. We know (and research in the USA shows[14]) that some menopausal autistic people simply avoid seeking healthcare or social care when they really need it. We recall one participant who said the 'NHS [National Health Service] is just absolute, just trauma,

I can't even go near it'.[15] Daisy also alluded to feeling suicidal in the context of her inability to access coordinated, holistic support for co-occurring, intersecting conditions.

This reminds us of that quote from Chapter 11 (page 116): 'I am the sum of my parts and any and all care I've received has fallen short because it's attempted to treat my parts separately if it considers them at all...'[16] You might recall, in the same chapter, that our autistic experts were highly aware that intersectional, marginalized aspects of their identity, like being queer, were unacknowledged and unsupported in menopause care. The high likelihood of co-occurring conditions, gender divergence, gender dysphoria or lifetime adversity and trauma – all of these on top of the unique way that an individual experiences their neurodivergence, and how it interacts with their menopause – is a reason why standard offerings may be inadequate and ill-fitting for autistic people, why person-centred, individualized support is imperative, and why key decision-makers need to find ways to make this happen as a matter of course.

Throughout this book, we've hopefully conveyed the significance of menopause (Part 1), why it might be especially challenging for neurodivergent people (Part 2), some of the difficulties they face (Part 3), and some of the ways they've coped (Part 4). As you saw in Chapters 15, 17 and this chapter, menopausal autistic people have often ended up going it alone. This is unacceptable, and on this note, we move to our concluding chapter, where we highlight what we'd like to see happen in terms of future support for autistic people before, during and after menopause.

Chapter 21

Conclusion

Looking to the future (where are we now and where do we need to go?)

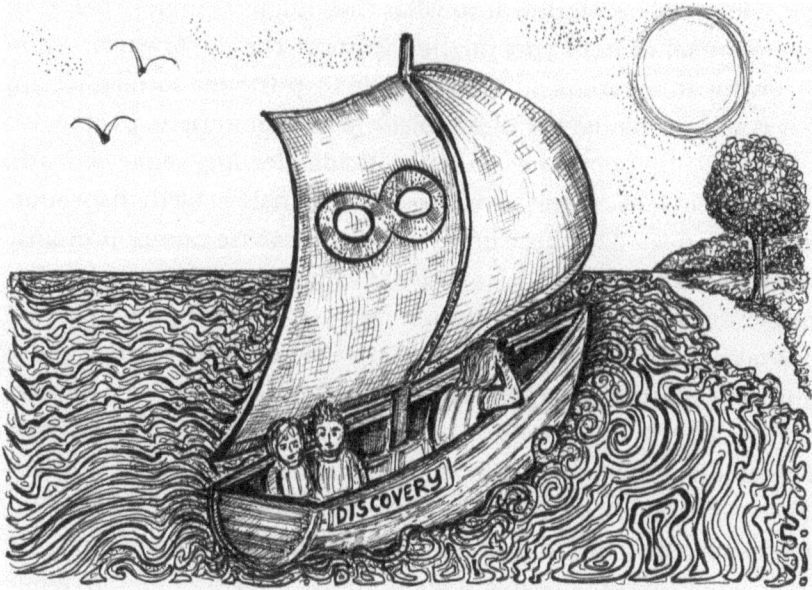

Thank you for coming on this journey with us. If you're autistic, we truly hope that reading this book has been, in the words of one person who wrote to us about our research, 'a light in a dark room' – revealing the very real and valid reasons why you might be struggling, providing reassurance that you're not alone, and comfort that there really is a way through.

The process of writing this book has been as much an illumination to us as we hope it has been for you. We have learnt so much from our experts, who have been tour-guides on what it is to experience an autistic menopause. We were honoured to hear their stories, rich with humour, wisdom and resilience, even while they expressed depths of despair and suffering. We've been staggered by their experiences that are undoubtedly shared by so many others, who may be unseen and unsupported, some unable to communicate their own story, and some lacking the vital explanation of a diagnosis which explains their lifelong struggles. The scale of unmet need is considerable when faced with these gaps in knowledge and understanding. How do we change this so more help and support is at hand?

We know that there are so many dedicated health and social care professionals doing their best in difficult circumstances. We hope that reading this book has given those who support or work with autistic people a window into what they might experience during menopause, to help you further support them. However, while receiving appropriate support remains a postcode lottery, we are not going to change the blunt, bleak facts that autistic people live shorter lives in poorer health, with suicide a leading cause of death, and autistic women and people assigned female at birth disproportionately affected by these negative outcomes.[1] We cannot presently link these facts to difficulties and inadequate support during menopause, but we hope that we have shown you the monumental toll it can take on health and wellbeing. There is no way to address these unmet needs without significant investment from key decision-makers who govern the provision and nature of health and social care. This book should serve as a call to action to policymakers in the UK and beyond. It's clear that one fundamental area of need is for accessible, inclusive and specific education about menopause for those whose experience might not fit the cookie-cutter mould. While our experts offered initial insights for change in Chapter 20, there is work to be done around learning from autistic people what other kinds of support they need before, during and after menopause; developing and evaluating evidence-based approaches in partnership with the autistic community; and finding systemic ways these can be delivered. Since provision of support fundamentally depends on identification of undiagnosed autistic people, this also highlights the need to address the 'avoidable and devastating'[2] crisis in waiting times for autism assessments in the UK. These are not trivial issues

– if you think back to Chapter 13, you'll see they may literally be a matter of life or death.

In the face of such challenges, it can be so difficult to know what you, the individual, can possibly do to help. You've started to do that already, in reading this book, and we would urge you to talk about menopause. Talk to the autistic people in your lives, or to each other if you're autistic. Talk to other professionals who might never have considered this area of unmet need. Talk to anyone who might have sway further up the chain of influence in health and social care. We need the issue of autistic menopause, and indeed neurodivergent, minority and marginalized menopauses more broadly, to gain the visibility that menopause as a whole has begun to have in the past decade. Autistic women and people assigned female at birth have been invisible for so long, and it's not been kind to their health and wellbeing.

Our last words must be to those autistic people going through menopause now, and those adapting to the new world on the other side. We hope you have found connection with our experts and their stories, and we hope that you'll find connection with other autistic people who understand the road you're walking. In this world, autistic people so often go through their lives feeling broken and deficient, indeed, being made to feel this way. The most important message we want to leave you with is Florence's words: 'You are worth it.' We know that these are just words on a page, but please believe that we imbue those words with our most heartfelt sentiments.

Yours,

Rachel and Julie

Resources

There are many social media groups (e.g. on Facebook) for autistic people and ADHDers going through menopause and for older individuals on the other side of menopause. We would encourage you to find these sources of connection.

To read our research, please see Rachel's site, which also includes a resources section linking you to further reading, podcasts and webinars on this topic: www.scienceonthespectrum.net

The National Autistic Society's page on autism and menopause, which includes a lot of useful help and support: www.autism.org.uk/advice-and-guidance/topics/physical-health/menopause

For people who identify as queer, transgender or other identities outside of the gender binary, with additional links to other minority kinds of menopause support:

- **Beyond Reflections**: https://beyond-reflections.org.uk
- **Queer Menopause**: www.queermenopause.com

Henpicked: Menopause in the Workplace Henpicked generously supported some of our research on autistic experiences of menopause, and their site includes a wealth of advice, tips, help and support: https://henpicked.net

My Menopause Centre, mentioned by our experts in Chapter 17: www.mymenopausecentre.com

People struggling with their mental health during menopause may wish to check out the following pages:

Mind: www.mind.org.uk/information-support/tips-for-everyday-living/menopause-and-mental-health

Articles in the **Balance Menopause Library**: www.balance-menopause.com/menopause-library

Unfortunately, there are no mental health resources specifically for autistic people (or autistic people at menopause), though you will find a few relevant resources gathered at Rachel's site, www.scienceonthespectrum.net. However, if you feel that your mental health is in a dangerous place during menopause, you might find it helpful to contact The Samaritans (call 116123, open 24/7) or the Shout crisis text line (text 85258, open 24/7).

Key points for professionals

- Autistic (neurodivergent) people may experience **menopausal symptoms as more severe** than non-autistic people. They are also more likely to have **complex mental and/or physical health conditions that might be worsened** by menopause.

- Autistic people might also experience **changes in features of their autism,** such as heightening of sensory sensitivities.

- **Take extra time to listen carefully to autistic people.** Different social communication styles mean that distress and emotion might be expressed differently, and they might sound unemotional even if they say they're struggling. People might also say they are 'OK' or 'fine' when asked, or that they understand something when they don't – often because they do not want to be a burden or 'bother' you. If individuals do verbally express distress or suicidal thoughts, **believe their words.** Autistic people find seeking help difficult, so they may be in extreme need by the time they reach out.

- **Adapt your communication style:**
  - Be concrete, clear and explicit, ideally providing information in a form they can take away, and giving extra time for explanations and questions.
  - Autistic people in distress often experience a regression in their communication skills as well as their abilities to cope with everyday life, so be mindful of this if you know the person well.

- Do not assume that patients can 'fill in the blanks' of brief explanations. Freely available information about menopause may not be accessible to them.
- Be wary of open questions. Autistic people sometimes struggle with recognizing their own emotions and bodily signals, and abstract questions like 'How do you feel?' Do whatever you can to reduce cognitive load. Some people might benefit from closed questions about possible symptoms, and may need descriptions of what symptoms might involve.

- **Adopt a trauma-informed and neurodiversity-affirmative approach**, helping autistic people to feel safe and accepted. This means seeing autism (and ADHD) as an equally valid way of being, not 'disordered' or 'deficient'.

- **Many older autistic people and ADHDers are undiagnosed**, including those at or approaching menopause. Late- and undiagnosed autistic people often have poorer mental health and more complex trauma. When you see individuals struggling with menopause, who may have a history of complex illness, relationship and employment difficulties, be mindful of possible autism and/or ADHD.

See these links for more guidance and resources.

- The **Autistic SPACE** framework for health and social care: www.magonlinelibrary.com/doi/full/10.12968/hmed.2023.0006 www.tandfonline.com/doi/full/10.1080/09503153.2024.2423405
- **ASPIRE Healthcare Toolkit**: https://researchautism.org/healthcaretoolkit
- **Choice Support** – guidance for social care: https://choicesupport.org.uk/about-us/what-we-do/supported-loving/supported-loving-toolkit/menopause-autism
- **Science on the Spectrum**: www.scienceonthespectrum.net/resources

Endnotes

INTRODUCTION
1   Davies J, Cooper K, Killick E, et al. Autistic identity: A systematic review of quantitative research. *Autism Research.* 2024;17:874–897.
2   Ibid.
      Pellicano E, den Houting J. Annual Research Review: Shifting from 'normal science' to neurodiversity in autism science. *Journal of Child Psychology and Psychiatry.* 2022;63(4):381–396.
3   Pellicano E, den Houting J. Annual Research Review: Shifting from 'normal science' to neurodiversity in autism science. *Journal of Child Psychology and Psychiatry.* 2022;63(4):381–96.

PART 1
1   Moseley RL, Druce T, Turner-Cobb J. 'When my autism broke': A qualitative study spotlighting autistic voices on menopause. *Autism.* 2020;24(6):1423–1437.
      Moseley RL, Druce T, Turner-Cobb JM. Autism research is 'all about the blokes and the kids': Autistic women breaking the silence on menopause. *British Journal of Health Psychology.* 2021;26(3):709–726.

CHAPTER 1
1   Harper JC, Phillips S, Biswakarma R, et al. An online survey of perimenopausal women to determine their attitudes and knowledge of the menopause. *Women's Health.* 2022;18:17455057221106890.
2   Moseley RL, Druce T, Turner-Cobb J. 'When my autism broke': A qualitative study spotlighting autistic voices on menopause. *Autism.* 2020;24(6):1423–1437.
      Moseley RL, Druce T, Turner-Cobb JM. Autism research is 'all about the blokes and the kids': Autistic women breaking the silence on menopause. *British Journal of Health Psychology.* 2021;26(3):709–726.
      Brady MJ, Jenkins CA, Gamble-Turner JM, Moseley RL, Janse van Rensburg M, Matthews RJ. 'A perfect storm': Autistic experiences of menopause and midlife. *Autism.* 2024;28(6):1405–1418.
      Jenkins C, Moseley R, Matthews R, Janse Van Rensburg M, Gamble-Turner J, Brady M. 'Struggling for years': An international survey on autistic experiences of menopause. *Neurodiversity.* 2024;2:27546330241299366.
      Karavidas M, de Visser RO. 'It's not just in my head, and it's not just irrelevant': Autistic negotiations of menopausal transitions. *Journal of Autism and Developmental Disorders.* 2022;52(3):1143–1155.
      Piper MA, Charlton RA. Common and unique menopause experiences among autistic and non-autistic people: A qualitative study. *Journal of Health Psychology.* 2024:13591053251316500.
3   Moseley RL, Druce T, Turner-Cobb JM. Autism research is 'all about the blokes and the kids': Autistic women breaking the silence on menopause. *British Journal of Health Psychology.* 2021;26(3):709–726.
      Piper MA, Charlton RA. Common and unique menopause experiences among autistic and non-autistic people: A qualitative study. *Journal of Health Psychology.* 2025 (online ahead of print):13591053251316500.

CHAPTER 2
1   Davis SR, Lambrinoudaki I, Lumsden M, et al. Menopause (Primer). *Nature Reviews: Disease Primers.* 2015;1:15004 (p.1).

2   Ellis S, Franks DW, Nielsen MLK, Weiss MN, Croft DP. The evolution of menopause in toothed whales. *Nature*. 2024;627(8004):579–585.
        Croft DP, Johnstone RA, Ellis S, et al. Reproductive conflict and the evolution of menopause in killer whales. *Current Biology*. 2017;27(2):298–304.

3   Wood BM, Negrey JD, Brown JL, et al. Demographic and hormonal evidence for menopause in wild chimpanzees. *Science*. 2023;382(6669):eadd5473.

4   Ellis S, Franks DW, Nielsen MLK, Weiss MN, Croft DP. The evolution of menopause in toothed whales. *Nature*. 2024;627(8004):579–585.

5   Croft DP, Johnstone RA, Ellis S, et al. Reproductive conflict and the evolution of menopause in killer whales. *Current Biology*. 2017;27(2):298–304.

6   Ibid.

7   Ellis S, Franks DW, Nielsen MLK, Weiss MN, Croft DP. The evolution of menopause in toothed whales. *Nature*. 2024;627(8004):579–585.

8   Tariq B, Phillips S, Biswakarma R, Talaulikar V, Harper JC. Women's knowledge and attitudes to the menopause: A comparison of women over 40 who were in the perimenopause, post menopause and those not in the peri or post menopause. *BMC Women's Health*. 2023;23(1):460.

9   Patel V, Ross S, Sydora BC. Assessing young adults' menopause knowledge to increase understanding of symptoms and help improve quality of life for women going through menopause; a student survey. *BMC Women's Health*. 2023;23(1):493.

10 Ambikairajah A, Walsh E, Cherbuin N. A review of menopause nomenclature. *Reproductive Health*. 2022;19(1):1–15.

11 Harlow SD, Gass M, Hall JE, et al. Executive summary of the Stages of Reproductive Aging Workshop + 10: Addressing the unfinished agenda of staging reproductive aging. *Climacteric*. 2012;15(2):105–114.

12 Ibid.

13 Davis SR, Lambrinoudaki I, Lumsden M, et al. Menopause (Primer). *Nature Reviews: Disease Primers*. 2015;1:15004.

14 Ibid.

15 Schoenaker DA, Jackson CA, Rowlands JV, Mishra GD. Socioeconomic position, lifestyle factors and age at natural menopause: A systematic review and meta-analyses of studies across six continents. *International Journal of Epidemiology*. 2014;43(5):1542–1562.

16 Davis SR, Lambrinoudaki I, Lumsden M, et al. Menopause (Primer). *Nature Reviews: Disease Primers*. 2015;1:15004.

17 Schoenaker DA, Jackson CA, Rowlands JV, Mishra GD. Socioeconomic position, lifestyle factors and age at natural menopause: A systematic review and meta-analyses of studies across six continents. *International Journal of Epidemiology*. 2014;43(5):1542–1562.

18 Ibid.

19 Ibid.

20 Ibid.

21 Davis SR, Lambrinoudaki I, Lumsden M, et al. Menopause (Primer). *Nature Reviews: Disease Primers*. 2015;1:15004.

22 Okeke T, Anyaehie U, Ezenyeaku C. Premature menopause. *Annals of Medical and Health Sciences Research*. 2013;3(1):90–95.

23 Davis SR, Lambrinoudaki I, Lumsden M, et al. Menopause (Primer). *Nature Reviews: Disease Primers*. 2015;1:15004.

24 Schmalenberger KM, Tauseef HA, Barone JC, et al. How to study the menstrual cycle: Practical tools and recommendations. *Psychoneuroendocrinology*. 2021;123:104895.
        Holt RI, Hanley NA. *Essential Endocrinology and Diabetes* (7th edition). John Wiley & Sons; 2021.

25 Barth C, Villringer A, Sacher J. Sex hormones affect neurotransmitters and shape the adult female brain during hormonal transition periods. *Frontiers in Neuroscience*. 2015;9:113668.
        Koebele SV, Ycaza Herrera A, Taylor CM, Barth C, Schwarz JM. Sex hormone fluctuations across the female lifespan: Mechanisms of action on brain structure, function, and behavior. *Frontiers in Behavioral Neuroscience*. 2022;16:964740.

26 Engler-Chiurazzi EB, Chastain WH, Citron KK, Lambert LE, Kikkeri DN, Shrestha SS. Estrogen, the peripheral immune system and major depression – a reproductive lifespan perspective. *Frontiers in Behavioral Neuroscience*. 2022;16:850623.

27 Bäckström T, Bixo M, Johansson M, et al. Allopregnanolone and mood disorders. *Progress in Neurobiology*. 2014;113:88–94.

28 Saunders KE, Hawton K. Suicidal behaviour and the menstrual cycle. *Psychological Medicine*. 2006;36(7):901–912.

29 Davis SR, Lambrinoudaki I, Lumsden M, et al. Menopause (Primer). *Nature Reviews: Disease Primers*. 2015;1:15004.

30 Hoyt LT, Falconi AM. Puberty and perimenopause: Reproductive transitions and their implications for women's health. *Social Science & Medicine*. 2015;132:103–112.

Brinton RD, Yao J, Yin F, Mack WJ, Cadenas E. Perimenopause as a neurological transition state. *Nature Reviews Endocrinology.* 2015;11(7):393-405.

31   Hoyt LT, Falconi AM. Puberty and perimenopause: Reproductive transitions and their implications for women's health. *Social Science & Medicine.* 2015;132:103-112.

32   Davis SR, Lambrinoudaki I, Lumsden M, et al. Menopause (Primer). *Nature Reviews: Disease Primers.* 2015;1:15004.

Fidecicchi T, Giannini A, Chedraui P, et al. Neuroendocrine mechanisms of mood disorders during menopause transition: A narrative review and future perspectives. *Maturitas.* 2024:108087.

CHAPTER 3

1   Brinton RD, Yao J, Yin F, Mack WJ, Cadenas E. Perimenopause as a neurological transition state. *Nature Reviews Endocrinology.* 2015;11(7):393-405.

2   Ibid.

3   Ibid.

4   Harper JC, Phillips S, Biswakarma R, et al. An online survey of perimenopausal women to determine their attitudes and knowledge of the menopause. *Women's Health.* 2022;18:17455057221106890.

5   Brinton RD, Yao J, Yin F, Mack WJ, Cadenas E. Perimenopause as a neurological transition state. *Nature Reviews Endocrinology.* 2015;11(7):393-405.

6   Deecher D, Dorries K. Understanding the pathophysiology of vasomotor symptoms (hot flushes and night sweats) that occur in perimenopause, menopause, and postmenopause life stages. *Archives of Women's Mental Health.* 2007;10:247-257.

7   Ibid.

8   Brinton RD, Yao J, Yin F, Mack WJ, Cadenas E. Perimenopause as a neurological transition state. *Nature Reviews Endocrinology.* 2015;11(7):393-405.

9   Ibid.

10   Reynolds F. Psychological responses to menopausal hot flushes: Implications of a qualitative study for counselling interventions. *Counselling Psychology Quarterly.* 1997;10(3):309-321.

11   Moseley RL, Druce T, Turner-Cobb JM. Unpublished supplementary data from 'Autism research is "all about the blokes and the kids": Autistic women breaking the silence on menopause.' (2021, *British Journal of Health Psychology*).

12   Davis SR, Lambrinoudaki I, Lumsden M, et al. Menopause (Primer). *Nature Reviews: Disease Primers.* 2015;1:15004.

13   Avis NE, Crawford SL, Greendale G, et al. Duration of menopausal vasomotor symptoms over the menopause transition. *JAMA Internal Medicine.* 2015;175(4):531-539.

14   Brinton RD, Yao J, Yin F, Mack WJ, Cadenas E. Perimenopause as a neurological transition state. *Nature Reviews Endocrinology.* 2015;11(7):393-405.

15   Ibid.

16   Gold EB, Colvin A, Avis N, et al. Longitudinal analysis of the association between vasomotor symptoms and race/ethnicity across the menopausal transition: Study of women's health across the nation. *American Journal of Public Health.* 2006;96(7):1226-1235.

17   Avis NE, Crawford SL, Greendale G, et al. Duration of menopausal vasomotor symptoms over the menopause transition. *JAMA Internal Medicine.* 2015;175(4):531-539.

18   Gold EB, Colvin A, Avis N, et al. Longitudinal analysis of the association between vasomotor symptoms and race/ethnicity across the menopausal transition: Study of women's health across the nation. *American Journal of Public Health.* 2006;96(7):1226-1235.

19   Ibid.

20   Brinton RD, Yao J, Yin F, Mack WJ, Cadenas E. Perimenopause as a neurological transition state. *Nature Reviews Endocrinology.* 2015;11(7):393-405.

21   El Khoudary SR, Greendale G, Crawford SL, et al. The menopause transition and women's health at midlife: A progress report from the Study of Women's Health Across the Nation (SWAN). *Menopause.* 2019;26(10):1213-1227.

Mosconi L, Berti V, Dyke J, et al. Menopause impacts human brain structure, connectivity, energy metabolism, and amyloid-beta deposition. *Scientific Reports.* 2021;11(1):10867.

Koebele SV, Bimonte-Nelson HA. The endocrine-brain-aging triad where many paths meet: Female reproductive hormone changes at midlife and their influence on circuits important for learning and memory. *Experimental Gerontology.* 2017;94:14-23.

Koebele SV, Mennenga SE, Hiroi R, et al. Cognitive changes across the menopause transition: A longitudinal evaluation of the impact of age and ovarian status on spatial memory. *Hormones and Behavior.* 2017;87:96-114.

22   Moseley RL, Druce T, Turner-Cobb JM. Autism research is 'all about the blokes and the kids': Autistic women breaking the silence on menopause. *British Journal of Health Psychology.* 2021;26(3):709-726.

23 El Khoudary SR, Greendale G, Crawford SL, et al. The menopause transition and women's health at midlife: A progress report from the Study of Women's Health Across the Nation (SWAN). *Menopause*. 2019;26(10):1213-1227.

24 Badawy Y, Spector A, Lee Z, Desai R. The risk of depression in the menopausal stages: A systematic review and meta-analysis. *Journal of Affective Disorders*. 2024;357:126-133.

25 Fidecicchi T, Giannini A, Chedraui P, et al. Neuroendocrine mechanisms of mood disorders during menopause transition: A narrative review and future perspectives. *Maturitas*. 2024;188:108087.

26 Avis NE, Crawford SL, Greendale G, et al. Duration of menopausal vasomotor symptoms over the menopause transition. *JAMA Internal Medicine*. 2015;175(4):531-539.
    Borkoles E, Reynolds N, Thompson DR, Ski CF, Stojanovska L, Polman RC. The role of depressive symptomatology in peri-and post-menopause. *Maturitas*. 2015;81(2):306-310.

27 Gold EB, Colvin A, Avis N, et al. Longitudinal analysis of the association between vasomotor symptoms and race/ethnicity across the menopausal transition: Study of women's health across the nation. *American Journal of Public Health*. 2006;96(7):1226-1235.

28 El Khoudary SR, Greendale G, Crawford SL, et al. The menopause transition and women's health at midlife: A progress report from the Study of Women's Health Across the Nation (SWAN). *Menopause*. 2019;26(10):1213-1227.

29 Ibid.

30 Brady MJ, Jenkins CA, Gamble-Turner JM, Moseley RL, Janse van Rensburg M, Matthews RJ. 'A perfect storm': Autistic experiences of menopause and midlife. *Autism*. 2024;28(6):1405-1418.

31 El Khoudary SR, Greendale G, Crawford SL, et al. The menopause transition and women's health at midlife: A progress report from the Study of Women's Health Across the Nation (SWAN). *Menopause*. 2019;26(10):1213-1227.

32 Verdonk P, Bendien E, Appelman Y. Menopause and work: A narrative literature review about menopause, work and health. *Work*. 2022;72(2):483-496.
    Rees M, Abernethy K, Bachmann G, et al. The essential menopause curriculum for healthcare professionals: A European Menopause and Andropause Society (EMAS) position statement. *Maturitas*. 2022;158:70-77.
    Gottardello D, Steffan B. Fundamental intersectionality of menopause and neurodivergence experiences at work. *Maturitas*. 2024;189:108107.

33 Bazeley A, Marren C, Shepherd A. *Menopause and the Workplace*. The Fawcett Society; 2022.

34 Brinton RD, Yao J, Yin F, Mack WJ, Cadenas E. Perimenopause as a neurological transition state. *Nature Reviews Endocrinology*. 2015;11(7):393-405.

35 El Khoudary SR, Greendale G, Crawford SL, et al. The menopause transition and women's health at midlife: A progress report from the Study of Women's Health Across the Nation (SWAN). *Menopause*. 2019;26(10):1213-1227.
    de Kruif M, Spijker A, Molendijk M. Depression during the perimenopause: A meta-analysis. *Journal of Affective Disorders*. 2016;206:174-180.

36 Harper JC, Phillips S, Biswakarma R, et al. An online survey of perimenopausal women to determine their attitudes and knowledge of the menopause. *Women's Health*. 2022;18:17455057221106890.

37 James DL, Larkey LK, Evans B, et al. Mechanisms of improved body composition among perimenopausal women practicing Meditative Movement: A proposed biobehavioral model. *Menopause*. 2023;30(11):1114-1123.
    Bondarev D, Laakkonen EK, Finni T, et al. Physical performance in relation to menopause status and physical activity. *Menopause*. 2018;25(12):1432-1441.

38 Steffan B, Potočnik K. Thinking outside Pandora's Box: Revealing differential effects of coping with physical and psychological menopause symptoms at work. *Human Relations*. 2023;76(8):1191-1225 (p.1213).

39 O'Reilly K, McDermid F, McInnes S, Peters K. 'I was just a shell': Mental health concerns for women in perimenopause and menopause. *International Journal of Mental Health Nursing*. 2024;33(3):693-702 (p.699).

CHAPTER 4

1   Avis NE, Crawford SL, Greendale G, et al. Duration of menopausal vasomotor symptoms over the menopause transition. *JAMA Internal Medicine*. 2015;175(4):531-539.
    Gold EB, Colvin A, Avis N, et al. Longitudinal analysis of the association between vasomotor symptoms and race/ethnicity across the menopausal transition: Study of women's health across the nation. *American Journal of Public Health*. 2006;96(7):1226-1235.

2   Harper JC, Phillips S, Biswakarma R, et al. An online survey of perimenopausal women to determine their attitudes and knowledge of the menopause. *Women's Health*. 2022;18:17455057221106890.

3   Huang DR, Goodship A, Webber I, et al. Experience and severity of menopause symptoms and effects on health-seeking behaviours: A cross-sectional online survey of community dwelling adults in the United Kingdom. *BMC Women's Health*. 2023;23(1):373.

Richard-Davis G, Singer A, King DD, Mattle L. Understanding attitudes, beliefs, and behaviors surrounding menopause transition: Results from three surveys. *Patient Related Outcome Measures*. 2022;13:273–286.

4   Gold EB, Colvin A, Avis N, et al. Longitudinal analysis of the association between vasomotor symptoms and race/ethnicity across the menopausal transition: Study of women's health across the nation. *American Journal of Public Health*. 2006;96(7):1226–1235.

5   Harper JC, Phillips S, Biswakarma R, et al. An online survey of perimenopausal women to determine their attitudes and knowledge of the menopause. *Women's Health*. 2022;18:17455057221106890.

6   Tariq B, Phillips S, Biswakarma R, Talaulikar V, Harper JC. Women's knowledge and attitudes to the menopause: A comparison of women over 40 who were in the perimenopause, post menopause and those not in the peri or post menopause. *BMC Women's Health*. 2023;23(1):460.

Patel V, Ross S, Sydora BC. Assessing young adults' menopause knowledge to increase understanding of symptoms and help improve quality of life for women going through menopause; a student survey. *BMC Women's Health*. 2023;23(1):493.

7   Martin-Key NA, Funnell EL, Spadaro B, Bahn S. Perceptions of healthcare provision throughout the menopause in the UK: A mixed-methods study. *npj Women's Health*. 2023;1(1):2.

Panay N, Ang SB, Cheshire R, et al. Menopause and MHT in 2024: Addressing the key controversies – an International Menopause Society White Paper. *South African General Practitioner*. 2024;5(3):119–134.

8   Harper JC, Phillips S, Biswakarma R, et al. An online survey of perimenopausal women to determine their attitudes and knowledge of the menopause. *Women's Health*. 2022;18:17455057221106890.

9   Ibid.

10 O'Reilly K, McDermid F, McInnes S, Peters K. An exploration of women's knowledge and experience of perimenopause and menopause: An integrative literature review. *Journal of Clinical Nursing*. 2023;32(15–16):4528–4540.

11 Moseley RL, Druce T, Turner-Cobb J. 'When my autism broke': A qualitative study spotlighting autistic voices on menopause. *Autism*. 2020;24(6):1423–1437.

Moseley RL, Druce T, Turner-Cobb JM. Autism research is 'all about the blokes and the kids': Autistic women breaking the silence on menopause. *British Journal of Health Psychology*. 2021;26(3):709–726.

Harper JC, Phillips S, Biswakarma R, et al. An online survey of perimenopausal women to determine their attitudes and knowledge of the menopause. *Women's Health*. 2022;18:17455057221106890.

Brady MJ, Jenkins CA, Gamble-Turner JM, Moseley RL, Janse van Rensburg M, Matthews RJ. 'A perfect storm': Autistic experiences of menopause and midlife. *Autism*. 2024;28(6):1405–1418.

Gottardello D, Steffan B. Fundamental intersectionality of menopause and neurodivergence experiences at work. *Maturitas*. 2024;189:108107.

12 Jermyn D. 'Everything you need to embrace the change': The 'menopausal turn' in contemporary UK culture. *Journal of Aging Studies*. 2023;64:101114.

13 Ibid.

14 Ibid.

Harper J, Keay N, Rowe F, Alstyne PV, Tariq S. The time has come for a UK-wide menopause education and support programme: InTune. *Women's Health*. 2024;20:17455057241277535.

15 Harper JC, Phillips S, Biswakarma R, et al. An online survey of perimenopausal women to determine their attitudes and knowledge of the menopause. *Women's Health*. 2022;18:17455057221106890.

Tariq B, Phillips S, Biswakarma R, Talaulikar V, Harper JC. Women's knowledge and attitudes to the menopause: A comparison of women over 40 who were in the perimenopause, post menopause and those not in the peri or post menopause. *BMC Women's Health*. 2023;23(1):460.

Ray E, Maybin JA, Harper JC. Perimenopausal women's voices: How does their period at the end of reproductive life affect wellbeing? *Post Reproductive Health*. 2023;29(4):201–221.

Hickey M, LaCroix AZ, Doust J, et al. An empowerment model for managing menopause. *The Lancet*. 2024;403(10430):947–957.

16 Ayers B, Forshaw M, Hunter MS. The impact of attitudes towards the menopause on women's symptom experience: A systematic review. *Maturitas*. 2010;65(1):28–36.

17 Ibid.

18 Crum AJ, Akinola M, Martin A, Fath S. The role of stress mindset in shaping cognitive, emotional, and physiological responses to challenging and threatening stress. *Anxiety, Stress, & Coping*. 2017;30(4):379–395.

19 Ibid.

20 Leventhal H, Phillips LA, Burns E. The Common-Sense Model of Self-Regulation (CSM): A dynamic framework for understanding illness self-management. *Journal of Behavioral Medicine.* 2016;39:935–946.
21 Ibid.
22 Leventhal H, Phillips LA, Burns E. The Common-Sense Model of Self-Regulation (CSM): A dynamic framework for understanding illness self-management. *Journal of Behavioral Medicine.* 2016;39:935–946.
      Leventhal H, Leventhal EA, Contrada RJ. Self-regulation, health, and behavior: A perceptual-cognitive approach. *Psychology and Health.* 1998;13(4):717–733.
      Leventhal H, Diefenbach M, Leventhal EA. Illness cognition: Using common sense to understand treatment adherence and affect cognition interactions. *Cognitive Therapy and Research.* 1992;16:143–163.
23 Hunter M, O'Dea I. Cognitive appraisal of the menopause: The menopause representations questionnaire (MRQ). *Psychology, Health and Medicine.* 2001;6(1):65–76.
      Pimenta F, Ramos MM, Silva CC, Costa PA, Maroco J, Leal I. Self-regulation model applied to menopause: A mixed-methods study. *Climacteric.* 2020;23(1):84–92.
24 Hunter M, O'Dea I. Cognitive appraisal of the menopause: The menopause representations questionnaire (MRQ). *Psychology, Health and Medicine.* 2001;6(1):65–76 (p.68).
25 Ibid.
26 Brown L, Brown V, Judd F, Bryant C. It's not as bad as you think: Menopausal representations are more positive in postmenopausal women. *Journal of Psychosomatic Obstetrics & Gynecology.* 2018;39(4):281–288.
27 Harper JC, Phillips S, Biswakarma R, et al. An online survey of perimenopausal women to determine their attitudes and knowledge of the menopause. *Women's Health.* 2022;18:17455057221106890.
      Tariq B, Phillips S, Biswakarma R, Talaulikar V, Harper JC. Women's knowledge and attitudes to the menopause: A comparison of women over 40 who were in the perimenopause, post menopause and those not in the peri or post menopause. *BMC Women's Health.* 2023;23(1):460.
      Ray E, Maybin JA, Harper JC. Perimenopausal women's voices: How does their period at the end of reproductive life affect wellbeing? *Post Reproductive Health.* 2023;29(4):201–221.
      Hickey M, LaCroix AZ, Doust J, et al. An empowerment model for managing menopause. *The Lancet.* 2024;403(10430):947–957.
28 Süss H, Ehlert U. Psychological resilience during the perimenopause. *Maturitas.* 2020;131:48–56.
29 Ibid.
30 Brown L, Hunter MS, Chen R, et al. Promoting good mental health over the menopause transition. *The Lancet.* 2024;403(10430):969–983.
31 Hunter M, O'Dea I. Cognitive appraisal of the menopause: The menopause representations questionnaire (MRQ). *Psychology, Health and Medicine.* 2001;6(1):65–76.
32 Stone AA, Schwartz JE, Broderick JE, Deaton A. A snapshot of the age distribution of psychological well-being in the United States. *Proceedings of the National Academy of Sciences.* 2010;107(22):9985–9990.
33 Ibid.
34 Lachman ME, Teshale S, Agrigoroaei S. Midlife as a pivotal period in the life course: Balancing growth and decline at the crossroads of youth and old age. *International Journal of Behavioral Development.* 2015;39(1):20–31.
35 Ibid.
36 Ibid.
37 Helpman L. On the stress of being a woman: The synergistic contribution of sex as a biological variable and gender as a psychosocial one to risk of stress-related disorders. *Neuroscience Biobehavioral Review.* 2023;150:105211.
38 Dickerson SS, Kemeny ME. Acute stressors and cortisol responses: A theoretical integration and synthesis of laboratory research. *Psychological Bulletin.* 2004;130(3):355–391.
39 Lachman ME, Teshale S, Agrigoroaei S. Midlife as a pivotal period in the life course: Balancing growth and decline at the crossroads of youth and old age. *International Journal of Behavioral Development.* 2015;39(1):20–31.
40 Dickerson SS, Kemeny ME. Acute stressors and cortisol responses: A theoretical integration and synthesis of laboratory research. *Psychological Bulletin.* 2004;130(3):355–391.
41 Lachman ME, Teshale S, Agrigoroaei S. Midlife as a pivotal period in the life course: Balancing growth and decline at the crossroads of youth and old age. *International Journal of Behavioral Development.* 2015;39(1):20–31.
42 Süss H, Ehlert U. Psychological resilience during the perimenopause. *Maturitas.* 2020;131:48–56.

43 Harper JC, Phillips S, Biswakarma R, et al. An online survey of perimenopausal women to determine their attitudes and knowledge of the menopause. *Women's Health.* 2022;18:17455057221106890.

44 Hoyt LT, Falconi AM. Puberty and perimenopause: Reproductive transitions and their implications for women's health. *Social Science & Medicine.* 2015;132:103–112.

Wells N, Lekies K. Nature and the life course: Pathways from childhood nature experiences to adult environmentalism. *Children Youth and Environments.* 2006;16(1):1–24.

45 Seeman TE, Singer B, Wilkinson CW, McEwen B. Gender differences in age-related changes in HPA axis reactivity. *Psychoneuroendocrinology.* 2001;26(3):225–240.

46 Herrera AY, Hodis HN, Mack WJ, Mather M. Estradiol therapy after menopause mitigates effects of stress on cortisol and working memory. *Journal of Clinical Endocrinology & Metabolism.* 2017;102(12):4457–4466.

Woods NF, Mitchell ES, Smith-Dijulio K. Cortisol levels during the menopausal transition and early postmenopause: Observations from the Seattle Midlife Women's Health Study. *Menopause.* 2009;16(4):708–718.

47 Arnot M, Emmott EH, Mace R. The relationship between social support, stressful events, and menopause symptoms. *PLoS One.* 2021;16(1):e0245444.

CHAPTER 5

1 Sapolsky RM. *Why Zebras Don't Get Ulcers: The Acclaimed Guide to Stress, Stress-Related Diseases and Coping.* Holt Paperbacks; 2004.

2 Slavich GM, Roos LG, Mengelkoch S, et al. Social Safety Theory: Conceptual foundation, underlying mechanisms, and future directions. *Health Psychology Review.* 2023;17(1):5–59.

McEwen BS, Gianaros PJ. Stress- and allostasis-induced brain plasticity. *Annual Review of Medicine.* 2011;62:431–445.

3 Suglia SF, Clausing ES, Shelton RC, et al. Cumulative stress across the life course and biological aging in adulthood. *Psychosomatic Medicine.* 2024;86(3):137–145.

Cuevas AG, Cole SW, Belsky DW, McSorley A-M, Shon JM, Chang VW. Multi-discrimination exposure and biological aging: Results from the midlife in the United States study. *Brain, Behavior, & Immunity – Health.* 2024;39:100774.

4 Suglia SF, Clausing ES, Shelton RC, et al. Cumulative stress across the life course and biological aging in adulthood. *Psychosomatic Medicine.* 2024;86(3):137–145.

5 Johnson J, Chaudieu I, Ritchie K, Scali J, Ancelin ML, Ryan J. The extent to which childhood adversity and recent stress influence all-cause mortality risk in older adults. *Psychoneuroendocrinology.* 2020;111:104492–104492.

6 O'Nions E, Lewer D, Petersen I, et al. Estimating life expectancy and years of life lost for autistic people in the UK: A matched cohort study. *Lancet Regional Health – Europe.* 2024;36:100776.

7 Cortés YI, Marginean V. Key factors in menopause health disparities and inequities: Beyond race and ethnicity. *Current Opinion in Endocrine and Metabolic Research.* 2022;26:100389.

8 Hoyt LT, Falconi AM. Puberty and perimenopause: Reproductive transitions and their implications for women's health. *Social Science & Medicine.* 2015;132:103–112.

Ramezani Tehrani F, Amiri M. The association between chronic diseases and the age at natural menopause: A systematic review. *Women & Health.* 2021;61(10):917–936.

9 Shanmugan S, Loughead J, Cao W, et al. Impact of tryptophan depletion on executive system function during menopause is moderated by childhood adversity. *Neuropsychopharmacology.* 2017;42(12):2398–2406.

10 Kapoor E, Okuno M, Miller VM, et al. Association of adverse childhood experiences with menopausal symptoms: Results from the Data Registry on Experiences of Aging, Menopause and Sexuality (DREAMS). *Maturitas.* 2021;143:209–215.

11 Shanmugan S, Loughead J, Cao W, et al. Impact of tryptophan depletion on executive system function during menopause is moderated by childhood adversity. *Neuropsychopharmacology.* 2017;42(12):2398–2406.

Shanmugan S, Satterthwaite TD, Sammel MD, et al. Impact of early life adversity and tryptophan depletion on functional connectivity in menopausal women: A double-blind, placebo-controlled crossover study. *Psychoneuroendocrinology.* 2017;84:197–205.

12 Beatty Moody DL, Brown C, Matthews KA, Bromberger JT. Everyday discrimination prospectively predicts inflammation across 7-years in racially diverse midlife women: Study of women's health across the nation. *Journal of Social Issues.* 2014;70(2):298–314.

Beatty Moody DL, Chang Y-F, Pantesco EJ, et al. Everyday discrimination prospectively predicts blood pressure across 10 years in racially/ethnically diverse midlife women: Study of women's health across the nation. *Annals of Behavioral Medicine.* 2019;53(7):608–620.

13 Avis NE, Crawford SL, Greendale G, et al. Duration of menopausal vasomotor symptoms over the menopause transition. *JAMA Internal Medicine.* 2015;175(4):531–539.

Gold EB, Colvin A, Avis N, et al. Longitudinal analysis of the association between vasomotor symptoms and race/ethnicity across the menopausal transition: Study of women's health across the nation. *American Journal of Public Health.* 2006;96(7):1226–1235.

14 Cohen S, Underwood LG, Gottlieb BH. *Social Support Measurement and Intervention: A Guide for Health and Social Scientists.* Oxford University Press; 2000.

15 Cohen S, Wills TA. Stress, social support, and the buffering hypothesis. *Psychological Bulletin.* 1985;98(2):310–357.
Turner-Cobb JM, Sephton SE, Koopman C, Blake-Mortimer J, Spiegel D. Social support and salivary cortisol in women with metastatic breast cancer. *Psychosomatic Medicine.* 2000;62(3):337–345.

16 Ayers B, Forshaw M, Hunter MS. The impact of attitudes towards the menopause on women's symptom experience: A systematic review. *Maturitas.* 2010;65(1):28–36.

17 Hayfield N, Moore H, Terry G. 'Friends? Supported. Partner? Not so much...': Women's experiences of friendships, family, and relationships during perimenopause and menopause. *Feminism & Psychology.* 2024;34(3):443–463.

18 Ibid.

19 Arnot M, Emmott EH, Mace R. The relationship between social support, stressful events, and menopause symptoms. *PLoS One.* 2021;16(1):e0245444.

20 Hayfield N, Moore H, Terry G. 'Friends? Supported. Partner? Not so much...': Women's experiences of friendships, family, and relationships during perimenopause and menopause. *Feminism & Psychology.* 2024;34(3):443–463.

21 Ibid.

22 Ibid.

23 Martin-Key NA, Funnell EL, Spadaro B, Bahn S. Perceptions of healthcare provision throughout the menopause in the UK: A mixed-methods study. *npj Women's Health.* 2023;1(1):2.

24 Ibid.

25 Ibid. p.6.

26 El Khoudary SR, Greendale G, Crawford SL, et al. The menopause transition and women's health at midlife: A progress report from the Study of Women's Health Across the Nation (SWAN). *Menopause.* 2019;26(10):1213–1227.

27 Hoyt LT, Falconi AM. Puberty and perimenopause: Reproductive transitions and their implications for women's health. *Social Science & Medicine.* 2015;132:103–112.

28 Falconi AM. Sex-Based Differences in the Determinants of Old Age Life Expectancy: The Influence of Perimenopause. *Biodemography and Social Biology.* 2017;63(1):54-70.

29 Fidecicchi T, Giannini A, Chedraui P, et al. Neuroendocrine mechanisms of mood disorders during menopause transition: A narrative review and future perspectives. *Maturitas.* 2024;188:108087.
Behrman S, Crockett C. Severe mental illness and the perimenopause. *BJPsych Bulletin.* 2023;48(6):364–370.

30 Hoyt LT, Falconi AM. Puberty and perimenopause: Reproductive transitions and their implications for women's health. *Social Science & Medicine.* 2015;132:103–112.

31 Behrman S, Crockett C. Severe mental illness and the perimenopause. *BJPsych Bulletin.* 2023;48(6):364–370.

32 O'Reilly K, McDermid F, McInnes S, Peters K. 'I was just a shell': Mental health concerns for women in perimenopause and menopause. *International Journal of Mental Health Nursing.* 2024;33(3):693–702.

33 Harper JC, Phillips S, Biswakarma R, et al. An online survey of perimenopausal women to determine their attitudes and knowledge of the menopause. *Women's Health.* 2022;18:17455057221106890 (p.10).

34 O'Reilly K, McDermid F, McInnes S, Peters K. 'I was just a shell': Mental health concerns for women in perimenopause and menopause. *International Journal of Mental Health Nursing.* 2024;33(3):693–702 (p.697).

35 *Suicides in England and Wales: 2022 Registrations.* Office for National Statistics; 2023.

36 Martin-Key NA, Funnell EL, Barker EJ, Bahn S. Examining suicidality in relation to the menopause: A systematic review. *PLOS Mental Health.* 2024;1(6):e0000161.

37 Fu X-L, Qian Y, Jin X-H, et al. Suicide rates among people with serious mental illness: A systematic review and meta-analysis. *Psychological Medicine.* 2023;53(2):351–361.

38 Hoyt LT, Falconi AM. Puberty and perimenopause: Reproductive transitions and their implications for women's health. *Social Science & Medicine.* 2015;132:103–112.

39 Ibid.

40 Barinas-Mitchel E, Duan C, Brooks M, et al. Cardiovascular disease risk factor burden during the menopause transition and late midlife subclinical vascular disease: Does race/ethnicity matter? *Journal of the American Heart Association.* 2020;9(4):e013876.

41 Jakubowski KP, Barinas-Mitchell E, Chang Y-F, Maki PM, Matthews KA, Thurston RC. The cardiovascular cost of silence: Relationships between self-silencing and carotid atherosclerosis in midlife women. *Annals of Behavioral Medicine.* 2022;56(3):282–290.

42 Ibid.

43 Bove R, Okai A, Houtchens M, et al. Effects of menopause in women with multiple sclerosis: An evidence-based review. *Frontiers in Neurology.* 2021;12:554375.
    Dias RCA, Kulak Junior J, Ferreira da Costa EH, Nisihara RM. Fibromyalgia, sleep disturbance and menopause: Is there a relationship? A literature review. *International Journal of Rheumatic Diseases.* 2019;22(11):1961–1971.
    Thomas N, Gurvich C, Huang K, Gooley PR, Armstrong CW. The underlying sex differences in neuroendocrine adaptations relevant to myalgic encephalomyelitis chronic fatigue syndrome. *Frontiers in Neuroendocrinology.* 2022;66:100995.

44 Dormire SL, Becker H, Lin C-J. Menopause healthcare for women with physical disabilities. *Nurse Practitioner.* 2006;31(6):42–50.

45 Lachman ME, Teshale S, Agrigoroaei S. Midlife as a pivotal period in the life course: Balancing growth and decline at the crossroads of youth and old age. *International Journal of Behavioral Development.* 2015;39(1):20–31.

PART 2

1 Brady MJ, Jenkins CA, Gamble-Turner JM, Moseley RL, Janse van Rensburg M, Matthews RJ. 'A perfect storm': Autistic experiences of menopause and midlife. *Autism.* 2024;28(6):1405–1418.
    Jenkins C, Moseley R, Matthews R, Janse Van Rensburg M, Gamble-Turner J, Brady M. 'Struggling for years': An international survey on autistic experiences of menopause. *Neurodiversity.* 2024;2:27546330241299366.

CHAPTER 6

1 Shamsalizadeh N, Rouhana N, Pierce CS, Swain MA. Formation of diverse meanings of menopause: An integrative literature review. *International Journal of Women's Health & Reproduction Sciences.* 2023;11(2):45–57.

CHAPTER 7

1 Stark E, Stacey J, Mandy W, Kringelbach ML, Happé F. Autistic cognition: Charting routes to anxiety. *Trends in Cognitive Science.* 2021;25(7):571–581.

2 Martin-Key NA, Funnell EL, Spadaro B, Bahn S. Perceptions of healthcare provision throughout the menopause in the UK: A mixed-methods study. *npj Women's Health.* 2023;1(1):2.
    Panay N, Ang SB, Cheshire R, et al. Menopause and MHT in 2024: Addressing the key controversies – an International Menopause Society White Paper. *South African General Practitioner.* 2024;5(3):119–134.

3 Moseley RL, Gregory NJ, Smith P, Allison C, Baron-Cohen S. A 'choice', an 'addiction', a way 'out of the lost': Exploring self-injury in autistic people without intellectual disability. *Molecular Autism.* 2019;10(1):1–23.

4 Brede J, Babb C, Jones C, et al. 'For me, the anorexia is just a symptom, and the cause is the autism': Investigating restrictive eating disorders in autistic women. *Journal of Autism and Developmental Disorders.* 2020;50:4280–4296.

5 Conner CM, Golt J, Righi G, Shaffer R, Siegel M, Mazefsky CA. A comparative study of suicidality and its association with emotion regulation impairment in large ASD and US census-matched samples. *Journal of Autism and Developmental Disorders.* 2020;50(10):3545–3560.

6 Nosek M, Kennedy HP, Gudmundsdottir M. Distress during the menopause transition: A rich contextual analysis of midlife women's narratives. *Sage Open.* 2012;2(3):2158244012455178.

7 Rapaport H, Clapham H, Adams J, Lawson W, Porayska-Pomsta K, Pellicano E. 'In a state of flow': A qualitative examination of autistic adults' phenomenological experiences of task immersion. *Autism in Adulthood.* 2024;6(3):362–373.

8 Kenny L, Remington A, Pellicano E. Everyday executive function issues from the perspectives of autistic adolescents and their parents: Theoretical and empirical implications. *Autism.* 2024;28(9):13623613231224093.

9 Rapaport H, Clapham H, Adams J, Lawson W, Porayska-Pomsta K, Pellicano E. 'I live in extremes': A qualitative investigation of autistic adults' experiences of inertial rest and motion. *Autism.* 2024;28(5):1305–1315 (p.1310).

10 Russell G, Kapp SK, Elliott D, Elphick C, Gwernan-Jones R, Owens C. Mapping the autistic advantage from the accounts of adults diagnosed with autism: A qualitative study. *Autism in Adulthood.* 2019;1(2):124–133.

11 Hwang YIJ, Foley K-R, Elley K, et al. Experiences of performing daily activities in middle-aged and older autistic adults: A qualitative study. *Journal of Autism and Developmental Disorders.* 2023;53(5):2037–2049.

12   Kenny L, Remington A, Pellicano E. Everyday executive function issues from the perspectives of autistic adolescents and their parents: Theoretical and empirical implications. *Autism.* 2024;28(9):13623613231224093.

13   MacLennan K, O'Brien S, Tavassoli T. In our own words: The complex sensory experiences of autistic adults. *Journal of Autism and Developmental Disorders.* 2022;52(7):3061-3075 (p.3068).

14   Sibeoni J, Massoutier L, Valette M, et al. The sensory experiences of autistic people: A metasynthesis. *Autism.* 2022;26(5):1032-1045.

15   Metz S. Stimming as a form of autistic aesthetic experience, neuroqueering landscape. *Ought: The Journal of Autistic Culture.* 2024;5(2):14.

16   Trevisan DA, Parker T, McPartland JC. First-hand accounts of interoceptive difficulties in autistic adults. *Journal of Autism and Developmental Disorders.* 2021;51(10):3483-3491.

17   Diwadkar VA, Murphy ER, Freedman RR. Temporal sequencing of brain activations during naturally occurring thermoregulatory events. *Cerebral Cortex.* 2014;24(11):3006-3013.

18   Reynolds F. Psychological responses to menopausal hot flushes: Implications of a qualitative study for counselling interventions. *Counselling Psychology Quarterly.* 1997;10(3):309-321.

19   Avis NE, Crawford SL, Greendale G, et al. Duration of menopausal vasomotor symptoms over the menopause transition. *JAMA Internal Medicine.* 2015;175(4):531-539.

20   Trevisan DA, Parker T, McPartland JC. First-hand accounts of interoceptive difficulties in autistic adults. *Journal of Autism and Developmental Disorders.* 2021;51(10):3483-3491.

21   Piper MA, Charlton RA. Common and unique menopause experiences among autistic and non-autistic people: A qualitative study. *Journal of Health Psychology.* 2025 (online ahead of print):13591053251316500.

22   Longhurst P, Aspell J, Todd J, Swami V. 'There's no separating my view of my body from my autism': A qualitative study of positive body image in autistic individuals. *Body Image.* 2024;48:101655.

23   Healy S, Pacanowski C, Kennedy L, Obrusnikova I. 'This cage that I'm stuck inside': Autistic adults' perceptions of weight management, body weight, and body image. *Autism.* 2021;25(7):1985-1998 (p.1990).

24   Brede J, Babb C, Jones C, et al. 'For me, the anorexia is just a symptom, and the cause is the autism': Investigating restrictive eating disorders in autistic women. *Journal of Autism and Developmental Disorders.* 2020;50:4280-4296.

25   Pellicano E, Fatima U, Hall G, et al. A capabilities approach to understanding and supporting autistic adulthood. *Nature Reviews Psychology.* 2022;1(11):624-639.

26   Han E, Scior K, Avramides K, Crane L. A systematic review on autistic people's experiences of stigma and coping strategies. *Autism Research.* 2022;15(1):12-26.

27   Crocker J, Park LE. The costly pursuit of self-esteem. *Psychological Bulletin.* 2004;130(3):392-414.

28   Brede J, Babb C, Jones C, et al. 'For me, the anorexia is just a symptom, and the cause is the autism': Investigating restrictive eating disorders in autistic women. *Journal of Autism and Developmental Disorders.* 2020;50:4280-4296.

29   Cage E, Di Monaco J, Newell V. Experiences of autism acceptance and mental health in autistic adults. *Journal of Autism and Developmental Disorders.* 2018;48(2):473-484.

30   Nguyen W, Ownsworth T, Nicol C, Zimmerman D. How I see and feel about myself: Domain-specific self-concept and self-esteem in autistic adults. *Frontiers in Psychology.* 2020;11:913.

31   Crocker J, Park LE. The costly pursuit of self-esteem. *Psychological Bulletin.* 2004;130(3):392-414.

32   Lamash L, Meyer S. Work-related self-efficacy and illness identity in adults with autism. *International Journal of Environmental Research and Public Health.* 2022;20(1):122.

33   Abe Y, Sirichokchatchawan W, Sangkomkamhang U, Satthapisit S, Maes M. Antenatal depressive symptoms are strongly predicted by the severity of pre-menstrual syndrome: Results of partial least squares analysis. *International Journal of Clinical Health Psychology Review.* 2023;23(2):100356.
   Flores-Ramos M, Heinze G, Silvestri-Tomassoni R. Association between depressive symptoms and reproductive variables in a group of perimenopausal women attending a menopause clinic in México City. *Archives of Women's Mental Health.* 2010;13:99-105.

34   Steward R, Crane L, Mairi Roy E, Remington A, Pellicano E. 'Life is much more difficult to manage during periods': Autistic experiences of menstruation. *Journal of Autism and Developmental Disorders.* 2018;48(12):4287-4292.

35   Ibid. p.4287.

36   Ibid. p.4291.

37   Gray LJ, Durand H. Experiences of dysmenorrhea and its treatment among allistic and autistic menstruators: A thematic analysis. *BMC Women's Health.* 2023;23(1):1-13 (p.7).

38   Bürger I, Erlandsson K, Borneskog C. Perceived associations between the menstrual cycle and attention deficit hyperactivity disorder (ADHD): A qualitative interview study exploring lived experiences. *Sexual & Reproductive Healthcare.* 2024;40:100975.

39   Stuart V, Kitson-Reynolds E. Autistic women's experiences of the antenatal, intrapartum and early postnatal periods. *British Journal of Midwifery.* 2024;32(4):180–188.

40   Ibid.

      Grant A, Griffiths C, Williams K, Brown A. 'It felt like I had an old fashioned telephone ringing in my breasts': An online survey of UK autistic birthing parents' experiences of infant feeding. *Maternal & Child Nutrition.* 2024;20(1):e13581.

41   Ward JH, Weir E, Allison C, Baron-Cohen S. Increased rates of chronic physical health conditions across all organ systems in autistic adolescents and adults. *Molecular Autism.* 2023;14(1):35.

      Liu S, Larsson H, Kuja-Halkola R, Lichtenstein P, Butwicka A, Taylor MJ. Age-related physical health of older autistic adults in Sweden: A longitudinal, retrospective, population-based cohort study. *Lancet Healthy Longevity.* 2023;4(7):e307–e315.

42   Ward JH, Weir E, Allison C, Baron-Cohen S. Increased rates of chronic physical health conditions across all organ systems in autistic adolescents and adults. *Molecular Autism.* 2023;14(1):35.

      Grant S, Norton S, Weiland R, Scheeren A, Begeer S, Hoekstra R. Autism and chronic ill health: An observational study of symptoms and diagnoses of central sensitivity syndromes in autistic adults. *Molecular Autism.* 2022;13(1):7.

43   Lai M-C. Mental health challenges faced by autistic people. *Nature Human Behaviour.* 2023;7(10):1620–1637.

44   Martini MI, Kuja-Halkola R, Butwicka A, et al. Sex differences in mental health problems and psychiatric hospitalization in autistic young adults. *JAMA Psychiatry.* 2022;79(12):1188–1198.

45   Lim GY, Tam WW, Lu Y, Ho CS, Zhang MW, Ho RC. Prevalence of depression in the community from 30 countries between 1994 and 2014. *Scientific Reports.* 2018;8(1):2861.

46   Newell V, Phillips L, Jones C, Townsend E, Richards C, Cassidy S. A systematic review and meta-analysis of suicidality in autistic and possibly autistic people without co-occurring intellectual disability. *Molecular Autism.* 2023;14(1):1–37.

47   Liu RT, Bettis AH, Burke TA. Characterizing the phenomenology of passive suicidal ideation: A systematic review and meta-analysis of its prevalence, psychiatric comorbidity, correlates, and comparisons with active suicidal ideation. *Psychological Medicine.* 2020;50(3):367–383.

      Nock MK, Borges G, Bromet EJ, et al. Cross-national prevalence and risk factors for suicidal ideation, plans and attempts. *British Journal of Psychiatry.* 2008;192(2):98–105.

48   Behrman S, Crockett C. Severe mental illness and the perimenopause. *BJPsych Bulletin.* 2023;48(6):364–370.

49   O'Reilly K, McDermid F, McInnes S, Peters K. 'I was just a shell': Mental health concerns for women in perimenopause and menopause. *International Journal of Mental Health Nursing.* 2024;33(3):693–702.

50   Henderson LM, St Clair M, Knowland V, Van Rijn E, Walker S, Gaskell M. Stronger associations between sleep and mental health in adults with autism: A UK Biobank study. *Journal of Autism and Developmental Disorders.* 2023;53(4):1543–1559.

51   Moseley RL, Druce T, Turner-Cobb J. 'When my autism broke': A qualitative study spotlighting autistic voices on menopause. *Autism.* 2020;24(6):1423–1437.

      Moseley RL, Druce T, Turner-Cobb JM. Autism research is 'all about the blokes and the kids': Autistic women breaking the silence on menopause. *British Journal of Health Psychology.* 2021;26(3):709–726.

      Brady MJ, Jenkins CA, Gamble-Turner JM, Moseley RL, Janse van Rensburg M, Matthews RJ. 'A perfect storm': Autistic experiences of menopause and midlife. *Autism.* 2024;28(6):1405–1418.

      Jenkins C, Moseley R, Matthews R, Janse Van Rensburg M, Gamble-Turner J, Brady M. 'Struggling for years': An international survey on autistic experiences of menopause. *Neurodiversity.* 2024;2:27546330241299366.

      Karavidas M, de Visser RO. 'It's not just in my head, and it's not just irrelevant': Autistic negotiations of menopausal transitions. *Journal of Autism and Developmental Disorders.* 2022;52(3):1143–1155.

      Piper MA, Charlton RA. Common and unique menopause experiences among autistic and non-autistic people: A qualitative study. *Journal of Health Psychology.* 2025 (online ahead of print):13591053251316500.

52   Harper JC, Phillips S, Biswakarma R, et al. An online survey of perimenopausal women to determine their attitudes and knowledge of the menopause. *Women's Health.* 2022;18:17455057221106890.

      O'Reilly K, McDermid F, McInnes S, Peters K. An exploration of women's knowledge and experience of perimenopause and menopause: An integrative literature review. *Journal of Clinical Nursing.* 2023;32(15-16):4528–4540.

53   Harper JC, Phillips S, Biswakarma R, et al. An online survey of perimenopausal women to determine their attitudes and knowledge of the menopause. *Women's Health.* 2022;18:17455057221106890.

Hayfield N, Moore H, Terry G. 'Friends? Supported. Partner? Not so much...': Women's experiences of friendships, family, and relationships during perimenopause and menopause. *Feminism & Psychology*. 2024;34(3):443–463.

54 Jones SC, Gordon CS, Akram M, Murphy N, Sharkie F. Inclusion, exclusion and isolation of autistic people: Community attitudes and autistic people's experiences. *Journal of Autism and Developmental Disorders*. 2022;52:1131–1142.

55 Stewart GR, Luedecke E, Mandy W, Charlton RA, Happé F. Experiences of social isolation and loneliness in middle-aged and older autistic adults. *Neurodiversity*. 2024;2:27546330241245529.

56 Doherty M, Neilson S, O'Sullivan J, et al. Barriers to healthcare and self-reported adverse outcomes for autistic adults: A cross-sectional study. *BMJ Open*. 2022;12(2):e056904.

57 Shaw SC, Carravallah L, Johnson M, et al. Barriers to healthcare and a 'triple empathy problem' may lead to adverse outcomes for autistic adults: A qualitative study. *Autism*. 2024;28(7):13623613231205629.

58 Hedley D, Uljarević M, Wilmot M, Richdale A, Dissanayake C. Brief report: Social support, depression and suicidal ideation in adults with autism spectrum disorder. *Journal of Autism and Developmental Disorders*. 2017;47:3669–3677.

Moseley R, Turner-Cobb J, Spahr CM, Shields GS, Slavich GM. Lifetime and perceived stress, social support, loneliness, and health in autistic adults. *Health Psychology*. 2021;40(8):556–568.

59 Hayfield N, Moore H, Terry G. 'Friends? Supported. Partner? Not so much...': Women's experiences of friendships, family, and relationships during perimenopause and menopause. *Feminism & Psychology*. 2024;34(3):443–463.

60 Pearson A, Rees J, Forster S. 'This was just how this friendship worked': Experiences of interpersonal victimization among autistic adults. *Autism in Adulthood*. 2022;4(2):141–150.

61 Quadt L, Williams G, Mulcahy J, et al. 'I'm trying to reach out, I'm trying to find my people': A mixed-methods investigation of the link between sensory differences, loneliness, and mental health in autistic and nonautistic adults. *Autism in Adulthood*. 2024;6(3):284–299 (p.295).

62 Bargiela S, Steward R, Mandy W. The experiences of late-diagnosed women with autism spectrum conditions: An investigation of the female autism phenotype. *Journal of Autism and Developmental Disorders*. 2016;46(10):3281–3294.

Kanfiszer L, Davies F, Collins S. 'I was just so different': The experiences of women diagnosed with an autism spectrum disorder in adulthood in relation to gender and social relationships. *Autism*. 2017;21(6):661–669.

63 Kanfiszer L, Davies F, Collins S. 'I was just so different': The experiences of women diagnosed with an autism spectrum disorder in adulthood in relation to gender and social relationships. *Autism*. 2017;21(6):661–669 (p.664).

64 Ljungberg M, Schön UK. Who cares? A scoping review about the experiences of parental caregivers of autistic adults. *Journal of Applied Research in Intellectual Disabilities*. 2023;36(5):929–939.

65 Shaw SC, Carravallah L, Johnson M, et al. Barriers to healthcare and a 'triple empathy problem' may lead to adverse outcomes for autistic adults: A qualitative study. *Autism*. 2024;28(7):13623613231205629.

66 Corden K, Brewer R, Cage E. A systematic review of healthcare professionals' knowledge, self-efficacy and attitudes towards working with autistic people. *Review Journal of Autism and Developmental Disorders*. 2022;9(3):386–399.

Grove R, Clapham H, Moodie T, Gurrin S, Hall G. 'Living in a world that's not about us': The impact of everyday life on the health and wellbeing of autistic women and gender diverse people. *Women's Health*. 2023;19:17455057231189542.

Radev S, Freeth M, Thompson ARJA. How healthcare systems are experienced by autistic adults in the United Kingdom: A meta-ethnography. *Autism*. 2024;28(9): 2166–2178.290

67 Dickerson SS, Kemeny ME. Acute stressors and cortisol responses: A theoretical integration and synthesis of laboratory research. *Psychological Bulletin*. 2004;130(3):355–391.

Slavich GM, Roos LG, Mengelkoch S, et al. Social Safety Theory: Conceptual foundation, underlying mechanisms, and future directions. *Health Psychology Review*. 2023;17(1):5–59.

68 Han E, Scior K, Avramides K, Crane L. A systematic review on autistic people's experiences of stigma and coping strategies. *Autism Research*. 2022;15(1):12–26.

Jones SC, Gordon CS, Akram M, Murphy N, Sharkie F. Inclusion, exclusion and isolation of autistic people: Community attitudes and autistic people's experiences. *Journal of Autism and Developmental Disorders*. 2022;52:1131–1142.

69 Pearson A, Rees J, Forster S. 'This was just how this friendship worked': Experiences of interpersonal victimization among autistic adults. *Autism in Adulthood*. 2022;4(2):141–150.

70 Fulton R, Reardon E, Kate R, Jones R. *Sensory Trauma: Autism, Sensory Difference and the Daily Experience of Fear*. Autism Wellbeing CIC; 2020.

71 Pellicano E, Fatima U, Hall G, et al. A capabilities approach to understanding and supporting autistic adulthood. *Nature Reviews Psychology.* 2022;1(11):624–639.

72 Rumball F, Happé F, Grey N. Experience of trauma and PTSD symptoms in autistic adults: Risk of PTSD development following DSM-5 and non-DSM-5 traumatic life events. *Autism Research.* 2020;13(12):2122–2132.

73 Geronimus A. *Weathering: The Extraordinary Stress of Ordinary Life on the Body in an Unjust Society.* Hachette UK; 2023.

74 Pellicano E, Fatima U, Hall G, et al. A capabilities approach to understanding and supporting autistic adulthood. *Nature Reviews Psychology.* 2022;1(11):624–639.

CHAPTER 8

1 Lachman ME, Teshale S, Agrigoroaei S. Midlife as a pivotal period in the life course: Balancing growth and decline at the crossroads of youth and old age. *International Journal of Behavioral Development.* 2015;39(1):20–31.

2 Radev S, Freeth M, Thompson AR. 'I'm not just being difficult... I'm finding it difficult': A qualitative approach to understanding experiences of autistic parents when interacting with statutory services regarding their autistic child. *Autism.* 2024;28(6):1394–1404.

3 Moseley RL, Druce T, Turner-Cobb JM. Unpublished supplementary data from 'Autism research is "all about the blokes and the kids": Autistic women breaking the silence on menopause.' (2021, *British Journal of Health Psychology*).

4 Brady MJ, Jenkins CA, Gamble-Turner JM, Moseley RL, Janse van Rensburg M, Matthews RJ. 'A perfect storm': Autistic experiences of menopause and midlife. *Autism.* 2024;28(6):1405–1418 (p.1411).

5 Moseley RL, Druce T, Turner-Cobb JM. Unpublished supplementary data from 'Autism research is "all about the blokes and the kids": Autistic women breaking the silence on menopause.' (2021, *British Journal of Health Psychology*).

6 Blackstone A. *Childfree by Choice: The Movement Redefining Family and Creating a New Age of Independence.* Penguin; 2019.

7 Ferland P, Caron SL. Exploring the long-term impact of female infertility: A qualitative analysis of interviews with postmenopausal women who remained childless. *Family Journal.* 2013;21(2):180–188.

8 Moseley RL, Druce T, Turner-Cobb JM. Unpublished supplementary data from 'Autism research is "all about the blokes and the kids": Autistic women breaking the silence on menopause.' (2021, *British Journal of Health Psychology*).

9 Piper MA, Charlton RA. Common and unique menopause experiences among autistic and non-autistic people: A qualitative study. *Journal of Health Psychology.* 2025 (online ahead of print):13591053251316500.

10 Moseley RL, Druce T, Turner-Cobb JM. Unpublished supplementary data from 'Autism research is "all about the blokes and the kids": Autistic women breaking the silence on menopause.' (2021, *British Journal of Health Psychology*).

11 Moseley RL, Druce T, Turner-Cobb JM. Autism research is 'all about the blokes and the kids': Autistic women breaking the silence on menopause. *British Journal of Health Psychology.* 2021;26(3):709–726.

12 Moseley RL, Druce T, Turner-Cobb JM. Unpublished supplementary data from 'Autism research is "all about the blokes and the kids": Autistic women breaking the silence on menopause.' (2021, *British Journal of Health Psychology*).

13 Ljungberg M, Schön UK. Who cares? A scoping review about the experiences of parental caregivers of autistic adults. *Journal of Applied Research in Intellectual Disabilities.* 2023;36(5):929–939.

14 *Outcomes for Disabled People in the UK: 2021.* Office for National Statistics; 2022.

15 Osborn E, Young R. Autistic and without a home: A systematic review and meta-ethnography of the presence and experiences of homelessness amongst autistic individuals. *Journal of Social Distress and Homelessness.* 2024;33(1):10–27.

16 Nicholas DB, Hedley D, Randolph JK, Raymaker DM, Robertson SM, Vincent J. An expert discussion on employment in autism. *Autism in Adulthood.* 2019;1(3):162–169.

17 Smethurst L, Thompson AR, Freeth M. 'I've absolutely reached rock bottom and have no energy': The lived experience of unemployed and underemployed autistic adults. *Autism in Adulthood.* 2024.

18 Bryson A, Conti G, Hardy R, Peycheva D, Sullivan A. The consequences of early menopause and menopause symptoms for labour market participation. *Social Science & Medicine.* 2022;293:114676.

Gomez-Leon M, Evandrou M, Falkingham J, Vlachantoni A. The dynamics of social care and employment in mid-life. *Ageing & Society.* 2019;39(2):381–408.

19 Moseley RL, Druce T, Turner-Cobb JM. Unpublished supplementary data from 'Autism research is "all about the blokes and the kids": Autistic women breaking the silence on menopause.' (2021, *British Journal of Health Psychology*).

20 Ibid.

21 Davies J, Matthews R, Romualdez AM, Pellicano E, Remington A. 'Retirement is one hell of a change': Autistic people's experiences of retiring. *Autism in Adulthood*. 2024 (online ahead of print).

22 Johnson MD, Somerville SD, Galambos NL, Krahn HJ. Stuck in the middle with you: Predictors of commitment in midlife. *International Journal of Behavioral Development*. 2020;44(3):273-278.

23 Currie H, Moger SJ. Menopause – understanding the impact on women and their partners. *Post Reproductive Health*. 2019;25(4):183-190.

24 Moseley RL, Druce T, Turner-Cobb JM. Autism research is 'all about the blokes and the kids': Autistic women breaking the silence on menopause. *British Journal of Health Psychology*. 2021;26(3):709-726 (p.717).

25 Moseley RL, Druce T, Turner-Cobb JM. Unpublished supplementary data from 'Autism research is "all about the blokes and the kids": Autistic women breaking the silence on menopause.' (2021, *British Journal of Health Psychology*).

26 Moseley RL, Druce T, Turner-Cobb JM. Autism research is 'all about the blokes and the kids': Autistic women breaking the silence on menopause. *British Journal of Health Psychology*. 2021;26(3):709-726.
    Brady MJ, Jenkins CA, Gamble-Turner JM, Moseley RL, Janse van Rensburg M, Matthews RJ. 'A perfect storm': Autistic experiences of menopause and midlife. *Autism*. 2024;28(6):1405-1418.

27 Davies J, Matthews R, Romualdez AM, Pellicano E, Remington A. 'Retirement is one hell of a change': Autistic people's experiences of retiring. *Autism in Adulthood*. 2024. DOI: 10.1089/aut.2023.0155
    Mansour H, Gillions A, Brown J, et al. 'It's designed for someone who is not me': A reflexive thematic analysis of the unmet healthcare support needs in UK autistic adults aged 65 years and over. *Autism*. 2024;29(3):13623613241291081.
    Aitken R, Berry K, Gowen E, Brown L. How do autistic adults experience ageing? A qualitative interview study. Unpublished manuscript, Open Science Framework, 2024.

28 Moseley RL, Druce T, Turner-Cobb JM. Unpublished supplementary data from 'Autism research is "all about the blokes and the kids": Autistic women breaking the silence on menopause.' (2021, *British Journal of Health Psychology*).

29 Brady MJ, Jenkins CA, Gamble-Turner JM, Moseley RL, Janse van Rensburg M, Matthews RJ. 'A perfect storm': Autistic experiences of menopause and midlife. *Autism*. 2024;28(6):1405-1418 (p.1411).

CHAPTER 9

1   Silberman S. *Neurotribes: The Legacy of Autism and the Future of Neurodiversity*. Avery; 2015.

2   American Psychiatric Association. *Diagnostic and Statistical Manual of Mental Disorders* (3rd edition). American Psychiatric Association; 1980.

3   Ibid.

4   American Psychiatric Association. *Diagnostic and Statistical Manual of Mental Disorders* (4th edition). Washington, DC: American Psychiatric Association; 1994.

5   American Psychiatric Association. *Diagnostic and Statistical Manual of Mental Disorders* (5th edition). American Psychiatric Association; 2013.

6   Lai M-C, Lin H-Y, Ameis SH. Towards equitable diagnoses for autism and attention-deficit/hyperactivity disorder across sexes and genders. *Current Opinion in Psychiatry*. 2022;35(2):90-100.

7   O'Nions E, Petersen I, Buckman JE, et al. Autism in England: Assessing underdiagnosis in a population-based cohort study of prospectively collected primary care data. *Lancet Regional Health – Europe*. 2023;29:100626.

8   Lai MC, Baron-Cohen S. Identifying the lost generation of adults with autism spectrum conditions. *Lancet Psychiatry*. 2015;2(11):1013-1027.

9   Moseley RL, Druce T, Turner-Cobb JM. Unpublished supplementary data from 'Autism research is "all about the blokes and the kids": Autistic women breaking the silence on menopause.' (2021, *British Journal of Health Psychology*).

10 Gellini H, Marczak M. 'I always knew I was different': Experiences of receiving a diagnosis of autistic spectrum disorder in adulthood – a meta-ethnographic systematic review. *Review Journal of Autism and Developmental Disorders*. 2023;11(3):620-639.

11 Moseley RL, Druce T, Turner-Cobb JM. Autism research is 'all about the blokes and the kids': Autistic women breaking the silence on menopause. *British Journal of Health Psychology*. 2021;26(3):709-726.

Gellini H, Marczak M. 'I always knew I was different': Experiences of receiving a diagnosis of autistic spectrum disorder in adulthood – a meta-ethnographic systematic review. *Review Journal of Autism and Developmental Disorders.* 2023;11(3):620–639.

12 Newell V, Phillips L, Jones C, Townsend E, Richards C, Cassidy S. A systematic review and meta-analysis of suicidality in autistic and possibly autistic people without co-occurring intellectual disability. *Molecular Autism.* 2023;14(1):1–37.

13 Moseley RL, Druce T, Turner-Cobb JM. Autism research is 'all about the blokes and the kids': Autistic women breaking the silence on menopause. *British Journal of Health Psychology.* 2021;26(3):709–726.

14 Ibid. p.718.

15 Ibid. p.715.

16 Gellini H, Marczak M. 'I always knew I was different': Experiences of receiving a diagnosis of autistic spectrum disorder in adulthood – a meta-ethnographic systematic review. *Review Journal of Autism and Developmental Disorders.* 2023;11(3):620–639.

17 Arnold SR, Huang Y, Hwang YI, Richdale AL, Trollor JN, Lawson L. 'The single most important thing that has happened to me in my life': Development of the Impact of Diagnosis Scale – Preliminary Revision. *Autism in Adulthood.* 2020;2(1):34–41.

18 Newell V, Phillips L, Jones C, Townsend E, Richards C, Cassidy S. A systematic review and meta-analysis of suicidality in autistic and possibly autistic people without co-occurring intellectual disability. *Molecular Autism.* 2023;14(1):1–37.

    Huang Y, Arnold SR, Foley KR, Lawson LP, Richdale AL, Trollor JN. Factors associated with age at autism diagnosis in a community sample of Australian adults. *Autism Research.* 2021;14(12):2677–2687.

    Mandy W, Midouhas E, Hosozawa M, Cable N, Sacker A, Flouri E. Mental health and social difficulties of late-diagnosed autistic children, across childhood and adolescence. *Journal of Child Psychology and Psychiatry.* 2022;63(11):1405–1414.

19 Cooper K, Russell AJ, Lei J, Smith LG. The impact of a positive autism identity and autistic community solidarity on social anxiety and mental health in autistic young people. *Autism.* 2023;27(3):848–857.

CHAPTER 10

1 Mencap. What is a learning disability? www.mencap.org.uk/learning-disability-explained/what-learning-disability. Accessed 27/10/2024.

2 Ibid.

3 Moseley RL, Druce T, Turner-Cobb J. 'When my autism broke': A qualitative study spotlighting autistic voices on menopause. *Autism.* 2020;24(6):1423–1437.

    Moseley RL, Druce T, Turner-Cobb JM. Autism research is 'all about the blokes and the kids': Autistic women breaking the silence on menopause. *British Journal of Health Psychology.* 2021;26(3):709–726.

4 Cummins C, Pellicano E, Crane L. Supporting minimally verbal autistic girls with intellectual disabilities through puberty: Perspectives of parents and educators. *Journal of Autism and Developmental Disorders.* 2018;50(7):2439–2448.

    Earle S, Ledger S, Newton V, Rouse L, Tilley E. Menstruation and learning disability across the life course: Using a two-part scoping exercise to co-produce research priorities. *British Journal of Learning Disabilities.* 2024;52(3):524–537.

5 Steward R, Crane L, Mairi Roy E, Remington A, Pellicano E. 'Life is much more difficult to manage during periods': Autistic experiences of menstruation. *Journal of Autism and Developmental Disorders.* 2018;48(12):4287–4292.

6 Earle S, Ledger S, Newton V, Rouse L, Tilley E. Menstruation and learning disability across the life course: Using a two-part scoping exercise to co-produce research priorities. *British Journal of Learning Disabilities.* 2024;52(3):524–537.

7 Langer-Shapland K, Minton SJ, Richards N. 'It should be more outspoken and not hushed away, not like put in a dark box': An interpretative phenomenological analysis of experiences of menopause voiced by women with learning disabilities. *British Journal of Learning Disabilities.* 2023;51(4):509–521.

8 Ibid. p.514.

9 Ibid. p.509.

10 Briggs P, Barsoum M, Soffe K. Challenges faced by women with learning disabilities, when they reach the menopause transition. *Post Reproductive Health.* 2023;29(2):113–118.

11 Bosco MCL. 'Bodies that never grow': How psychiatric understanding of autism spectrum disorders affects autistic people's bodily experience of gender, ageing, and sexual desire. *Journal of Aging Studies.* 2023;64:101101.

    Graham Holmes L, Ames JL, Massolo ML, Nunez DM, Croen LA. Improving the sexual and reproductive health and health care of autistic people. *Pediatrics.* 2022;149:e2020049437J.

12 Irvine B, Elise F, Brinkert J, et al. 'A storm of post-it notes': Experiences of perceptual capacity in autism and ADHD. *Neurodiversity.* 2024;2:27546330241229004 (p.9).

13 Irvine B, Elise F, Brinkert J, et al. 'A storm of post-it notes': Experiences of perceptual capacity in autism and ADHD. *Neurodiversity.* 2024;2:27546330241229004.

14 Dodson W. Secrets of your ADHD brain. ADDitude. 2022; www.additudemag.com/secrets-of-the-adhd-brain/?srsltid=AfmBOooCTvE1orX1o-rMzWE5ruBOZIjaqS9fIEuhLxnZCcmrwobsB fPI. Accessed 03/07/2025.

15 Loyer Carbonneau M, Demers M, Bigras M, Guay M-C. Meta-analysis of sex differences in ADHD symptoms and associated cognitive deficits. *Journal of Attention Disorders.* 2021;25(12):1640–1656.

16 Redshaw R, McCormack L. 'Being ADHD': A qualitative study. *Advances in Neurodevelopmental Disorders.* 2022;6(1):20–28 (p.23).

17 Nordby ES, Guribye F, Nordgreen T, Lundervold AJ. Silver linings of ADHD: A thematic analysis of adults' positive experiences with living with ADHD. *BMJ Open.* 2023;13(10):e072052.

18 Redshaw R, McCormack L. 'Being ADHD': A qualitative study. *Advances in Neurodevelopmental Disorders.* 2022;6(1):20–28 (p.24).

19 Irvine B, Elise F, Brinkert J, et al. 'A storm of post-it notes': Experiences of perceptual capacity in autism and ADHD. *Neurodiversity.* 2024;2:27546330241229004.

 Redshaw R, McCormack L. 'Being ADHD': A qualitative study. *Advances in Neurodevelopmental Disorders.* 2022;6(1):20–28.

 Bertilsdotter Rosqvist H, Hultman L, Österborg Wiklund S, Nygren A, Storm P, Sandberg G. Intensity and variable attention: Counter narrating ADHD, from ADHD deficits to ADHD difference. *British Journal of Social Work.* 2023;53(8):3647–3664.

 Schippers LM, Horstman LI, Velde Hvd, et al. A qualitative and quantitative study of self-reported positive characteristics of individuals with ADHD. *Frontiers in Psychiatry.* 2022;13:922788.

20 Dodson W. Secrets of your ADHD brain. ADDitude. 2022; www.additudemag.com/secrets-of-the-adhd-brain/?srsltid=AfmBOooCTvE1orX1o-rMzWE5ruBOZIjaqS9fIEuhLxnZCcmrwobsB fPI. Accessed 03/07/2025.

21 Antshel KM, Russo N. Autism spectrum disorders and ADHD: Overlapping phenomenology, diagnostic issues, and treatment considerations. *Current Psychiatry Reports.* 2019;21(5):1–11.

22 Schippers LM, Horstman LI, Velde Hvd, et al. A qualitative and quantitative study of self-reported positive characteristics of individuals with ADHD. *Frontiers in Psychiatry.* 2022;13:922788.

23 Rafi H, Murray R, Delavari F, et al. Neural basis of internal attention in adults with pure and comorbid ADHD. *Journal of Attention Disorders.* 2023;27(4):423–436.

24 Dodson WW, Modestino EJ, Ceritoğlu HT, Zayed B. Rejection sensitivity dysphoria in attention-deficit/hyperactivity disorder: A case series. *Neurology.* 2024;7:23–30.

25 Visser MJ, Peters RM, Luman M. Understanding ADHD-related stigma: A gender analysis of young adults and key stakeholder perspectives. *Neurodiversity.* 2024;2:27546330241274664.

26 Lai M-C, Lin H-Y, Ameis SH. Towards equitable diagnoses for autism and attention-deficit/hyperactivity disorder across sexes and genders. *Current Opinion in Psychiatry.* 2022;35(2):90–100.

27 Redshaw R, McCormack L. 'Being ADHD': A qualitative study. *Advances in Neurodevelopmental Disorders.* 2022;6(1):20–28.

28 Antoniou E, Rigas N, Orovou E, Papatrechas A, Sarella A. ADHD symptoms in females of childhood, adolescent, reproductive and menopause period. *Materia Socio-Medica.* 2021;33(2):114–118.

 Camara B, Padoin C, Bolea B. Relationship between sex hormones, reproductive stages and ADHD: A systematic review. *Archives of Women's Mental Health.* 2021;25(1):1–8.

29 ADDitude. ADHD impairment peaks in menopause, according to ADDitude reader survey. 2024; www.additudemag.com/menopause-symptoms-adhd-survey. Accessed 28/10/2024.

30 'Without perimenopause, I might not have realised I have ADHD'. Dr Louise Newson. 2022; www.balance-menopause.com/menopause-library/menopause-and-adhd. Accessed 03/07/2025.

31 Rong Y, Yang C-J, Jin Y, Wang Y. Prevalence of attention-deficit/hyperactivity disorder in individuals with autism spectrum disorder: A meta-analysis. *Research in Autism Spectrum Disorders.* 2021;83:101759.

32 Lebeña A, Faresjö Å, Faresjö T, Ludvigsson J. Clinical implications of ADHD, ASD, and their co-occurrence in early adulthood – the prospective ABIS-study. *BMC Psychiatry.* 2023;23(1):851.

 Yerys BE, McQuaid GA, Lee NR, Wallace GL. Co-occurring ADHD symptoms in autistic adults are associated with less independence in daily living activities and lower subjective quality of life. *Autism in Adulthood.* 2022;26(8):2188–2195.

33 Moseley RL, Druce T, Turner-Cobb JM. Autism research is 'all about the blokes and the kids': Autistic women breaking the silence on menopause. *British Journal of Health Psychology.* 2021;26(3):709–726.

34 Hargitai LD, Livingston LA, Waldren LH, Robinson R, Jarrold C, Shah P. Attention-deficit hyperactivity disorder traits are a more important predictor of internalising problems than autistic traits. *Scientific Reports.* 2023;13(1):31.

CHAPTER 11

1   Intersectionality. 2025; www.merriam-webster.com/dictionary/intersectionality. Accessed 14/01/2025.
2   Mason D. Healthcare barriers, what about older age? A comment on Malik-Soni et al. *Pediatric Research.* 2022;91(5):1025–1027.
3   Grove R, Clapham H, Moodie T, Gurrin S, Hall G. 'Living in a world that's not about us': The impact of everyday life on the health and wellbeing of autistic women and gender diverse people. *Women's Health.* 2023;19:17455057231189542.
4   Fannin DK, Williams EDG, Fuller M, et al. Unpacking the prevalence: A warning against overstating the recently narrowed gap for Black autistic youth. *Autism Research.* 2024;17(6):1072–1082.
    Jones DR, Mandell DS. To address racial disparities in autism research, we must think globally, act locally. *Autism.* 2020;24(7):1587–1589.
5   Wallace-Watkin C, Sigafoos J, Waddington H. Barriers and facilitators for obtaining support services among underserved families with an autistic child: A systematic qualitative review. *Autism.* 2023;27(3):588–601.
    Malone KM, Pearson JN, Palazzo KN, Manns LD, Rivera AQ, Mason Martin DL. The scholarly neglect of Black autistic adults in autism research. *Autism in Adulthood.* 2022;4(4):271–280.
6   Davis AM, Smith E, Yang X, Wright R. Exploring racial discrimination, disability discrimination, and perception of the future among Black-identifying emerging adults with and without autism in the United States: A mixed-methods descriptive study. *Journal of Child & Adolescent Trauma.* 2024;17(4):1019–1034.
7   Davis A, Solomon M, Belcher H. Examination of race and autism intersectionality among African American/Black young adults. *Autism in Adulthood.* 2022;4(4):306–314.
8   Cohen SR, Joseph K, Levinson S, Blacher J, Eisenhower A. 'My autism is my own': Autistic identity and intersectionality in the school context. *Autism in Adulthood.* 2022;4(4):315–327 (p.322).
9   Roberts J. Ableism, code-switching, and camouflaging: A letter to the editor on Gerlach-Houck and DeThorne (2023). *Language, Speech, and Hearing Services in Schools.* 2024;55(1):217–223.
10 Burkett C. 'Autistic while black': How autism amplifies stereotypes. The Transmitter. 2020, 21 January; www.thetransmitter.org/spectrum/autistic-while-black-how-autism-amplifies-stereotypes. Accessed 03/07/2025.
11 Nelson T. *'Before People See the Autism, They See My Race': An Intersectional Exploration of the Lived Experiences of Masking and Camouflaging Black Autistic Girls in UK Education Using IPA and DisCrit.* University of Essex & Tavistock and Portman NHS Foundation Trust; 2024.
12 Cortés YI, Marginean V. Key factors in menopause health disparities and inequities: Beyond race and ethnicity. *Current Opinion in Endocrine and Metabolic Research.* 2022;26:100389.
13 Ibid.
14 Ibid.
    Akpan P. Why research and conversation about menopause is letting down Black and Asian people. *Good Housekeeping.* 2021, 16 February.
    Bouzy J, Brunelle J, Cohen D, Condat A. Transidentities and autism spectrum disorder: A systematic review. *Psychiatry Research.* 2023;323:115176.
15 Bouzy J, Brunelle J, Cohen D, Condat A. Transidentities and autism spectrum disorder: A systematic review. *Psychiatry Research.* 2023;323:115176.
    Warrier V, Greenberg DM, Weir E, et al. Elevated rates of autism, other neurodevelopmental and psychiatric diagnoses, and autistic traits in transgender and gender-diverse individuals. *Nature Communications.* 2020;11(1):3959.
    Weir E, Allison C, Baron-Cohen S. The sexual health, orientation, and activity of autistic adolescents and adults. *Autism Research.* 2021;14(11):2342–2354.
16 Stonewall. List of LGBTQ+ terms. www.stonewall.org.uk/resources/list-lgbtq-terms. Accessed 27/10/2024.
17 Stonewall. LGBTQ+ facts and figures. www.stonewall.org.uk/resources/lgbtq-facts-and-figures. Accessed 14/01/2025.
18 Cheung A, Nolan B, Zwickl S. Transgender health and the impact of aging and menopause. *Climacteric.* 2023;26(3):256–262.
    Glyde T. LGBTQIA+ menopause: Room for improvement. *Lancet Child Adolescent Health.* 2022;400(10363):1578–1579.
19 Cheung A, Nolan B, Zwickl S. Transgender health and the impact of aging and menopause. *Climacteric.* 2023;26(3):256–262.

Glyde T. LGBTQIA+ menopause: Room for improvement. *Lancet Child Adolescent Health.* 2022;400(10363):1578–1579.

20   Thomas SD, King R, Murphy M, Dempsey M. Demographic factors associated with health-care avoidance and delay in the transgender population: Findings from a systematic review. *Dialogues in Health.* 2023;3:100159.

21   Bruce H, Munday K, Kapp SK. Exploring the experiences of autistic transgender and non-binary adults in seeking gender identity health care. *Autism in Adulthood.* 2023;5(2):191–203.
Wallisch A, Boyd BA, Hall JP, et al. Health care disparities among autistic LGBTQ+ people. *Autism in Adulthood.* 2023;5(2):165–174.

22   Brady MJ, Jenkins CA, Gamble-Turner JM, Moseley RL, Janse van Rensburg M, Matthews RJ. 'A perfect storm': Autistic experiences of menopause and midlife. *Autism.* 2024;28(6):1405–1418 (p.1410).

23   Malone KM, Pearson JN, Palazzo KN, Manns LD, Rivera AQ, Mason Martin DL. The scholarly neglect of Black autistic adults in autism research. *Autism in Adulthood.* 2022;4(4):271–280 (p.273).

CHAPTER 12

1   Groenman AP, Torenvliet C, Radhoe TA, Agelink van Rentergem JA, Geurts HM. Menstruation and menopause in autistic adults: Periods of importance? *Autism.* 2022;26(6):1563–1572.
Charlton RA, Happé F, Shand A, Mandy W, Stewart G. Self-reported psychological, somatic and vasomotor symptoms at different stages of the menopause for autistic and non-autistic people. *Journal of Women's Health.* 2025;34(5):622–634.

2   Charlton RA, Happé F, Shand A, Mandy W, Stewart G. Self-reported psychological, somatic and vasomotor symptoms at different stages of the menopause for autistic and non-autistic people. *Journal of Women's Health.* 2025;34(5):622–634.

3   Moseley RL, Druce T, Turner-Cobb JM. Autism research is 'all about the blokes and the kids': Autistic women breaking the silence on menopause. *British Journal of Health Psychology.* 2021;26(3):709–726.
Jenkins C, Moseley R, Matthews R, Janse Van Rensburg M, Gamble-Turner J, Brady M. 'Struggling for years': An international survey on autistic experiences of menopause. *Neurodiversity.* 2024;2:27546330241299366.

4   Moseley RL, Druce T, Turner-Cobb JM. Unpublished supplementary data from 'Autism research is "all about the blokes and the kids": Autistic women breaking the silence on menopause.' (2021, *British Journal of Health Psychology*).

5   Steward R, Crane L, Mairi Roy E, Remington A, Pellicano E. 'Life is much more difficult to manage during periods': Autistic experiences of menstruation. *Journal of Autism and Developmental Disorders.* 2018;48(12):4287–4292.
Gray LJ, Durand H. Experiences of dysmenorrhea and its treatment among allistic and autistic menstruators: A thematic analysis. *BMC Women's Health.* 2023;23(1):1–13.

6   Moseley RL, Druce T, Turner-Cobb JM. Unpublished supplementary data from 'Autism research is "all about the blokes and the kids": Autistic women breaking the silence on menopause.' (2021, *British Journal of Health Psychology*).

7   Piper MA, Charlton RA. Common and unique menopause experiences among autistic and non-autistic people: A qualitative study. *Journal of Health Psychology.* 2025 (online ahead of print):13591053251316500.

8   Greendale GA, Sternfeld B, Huang M, et al. Changes in body composition and weight during the menopause transition. *JCI Insight.* 2019;4(5):e124865.

9   Liu S, Larsson H, Kuja-Halkola R, Lichtenstein P, Butwicka A, Taylor MJ. Age-related physical health of older autistic adults in Sweden: A longitudinal, retrospective, population-based cohort study. *Lancet Healthy Longevity.* 2023;4(7):e307–e315.

10 Moseley RL, Druce T, Turner-Cobb J. 'When my autism broke': A qualitative study spotlighting autistic voices on menopause. *Autism.* 2020;24(6):1423–1437.
Moseley RL, Druce T, Turner-Cobb JM. Autism research is 'all about the blokes and the kids': Autistic women breaking the silence on menopause. *British Journal of Health Psychology.* 2021;26(3):709–726.
Brady MJ, Jenkins CA, Gamble-Turner JM, Moseley RL, Janse van Rensburg M, Matthews RJ. 'A perfect storm': Autistic experiences of menopause and midlife. *Autism.* 2024;28(6):1405–1418.

11 Weir E, Allison C, Warrier V, Baron-Cohen S. Increased prevalence of non-communicable physical health conditions among autistic adults. *Autism.* 2021;25(3):681–694.

12 Moseley RL, Druce T, Turner-Cobb JM. Autism research is 'all about the blokes and the kids': Autistic women breaking the silence on menopause. *British Journal of Health Psychology.* 2021;26(3):709–726.

CHAPTER 13

1   Nock MK, Wedig MM, Holmberg EB, Hooley JM. The emotion reactivity scale: Development, evaluation, and relation to self-injurious thoughts and behaviors. *Behavioral Therapy.* 2008;39(2):107–116.

2   Herrera AY, Hodis HN, Mack WJ, Mather M. Estradiol therapy after menopause mitigates effects of stress on cortisol and working memory. *Journal of Clinical Endocrinology & Metabolism.* 2017;102(12):4457–4466.
    Woods NF, Mitchell ES, Smith-Dijulio K. Cortisol levels during the menopausal transition and early postmenopause: Observations from the Seattle Midlife Women's Health Study. *Menopause.* 2009;16(4):708–718.
    Albert KM, Newhouse PA. Estrogen, stress, and depression: Cognitive and biological interactions. *Annual Review of Clinical Psychology.* 2019;15(1):399–423.

3   Beck KB, MacKenzie KT, Kumar T, et al. 'The world's really not set up for the neurodivergent person': Understanding emotion dysregulation from the perspective of autistic adults. *Autism in Adulthood.* 2024.
    Lewis LF, Stevens K. The lived experience of meltdowns for autistic adults. *Autism.* 2023;27(6):1817–1825.

4   Lewis LF, Stevens K. The lived experience of meltdowns for autistic adults. *Autism.* 2023;27(6):1817–1825 (p.1821).

5   Moseley RL, Druce T, Turner-Cobb JM. Autism research is 'all about the blokes and the kids': Autistic women breaking the silence on menopause. *British Journal of Health Psychology.* 2021;26(3):709–726.

6   Ibid.

7   Groenman AP, Torenvliet C, Radhoe TA, Agelink van Rentergem JA, Geurts HM. Menstruation and menopause in autistic adults: Periods of importance? *Autism.* 2022;26(6):1563–1572.
    Charlton RA, Happé F, Shand A, Mandy W, Stewart G. Self-reported psychological, somatic and vasomotor symptoms at different stages of the menopause for autistic and non-autistic people. *Journal of Women's Health.* 2025;34(5):622–634.

8   Angel L, Ailey SH, Delaney KR, Mohr L. Presentation of depressive symptoms in autism spectrum disorders. *Western Journal of Nursing Research.* 2023;45(9):854–861.

9   Brown CM, Newell V, Sahin E, Hedley D. Updated systematic review of suicide in autism: 2018–2024. *Current Developmental Disorders Reports.* 2024;11(4):225–256.

10 Moseley RL, Druce T, Turner-Cobb JM. Autism research is 'all about the blokes and the kids': Autistic women breaking the silence on menopause. *British Journal of Health Psychology.* 2021;26(3):709–726.
    Brady MJ, Jenkins CA, Gamble-Turner JM, Moseley RL, Janse van Rensburg M, Matthews RJ. 'A perfect storm': Autistic experiences of menopause and midlife. *Autism.* 2024;28(6):1405–1418.

11 Moseley RL, Druce T, Turner-Cobb JM. Unpublished supplementary data from 'Autism research is "all about the blokes and the kids": Autistic women breaking the silence on menopause.' (2021, *British Journal of Health Psychology*).

12 Moseley RL, Druce T, Turner-Cobb JM. Autism research is 'all about the blokes and the kids': Autistic women breaking the silence on menopause. *British Journal of Health Psychology.* 2021;26(3):709–726 (p.716).

CHAPTER 14

1   Gottardello D, Steffan B. Fundamental intersectionality of menopause and neurodivergence experiences at work. *Maturitas.* 2024;189:108107.
    ADDitude. ADHD impairment peaks in menopause, according to ADDitude reader survey. 2024; www.additudemag.com/menopause-symptoms-adhd-survey. Accessed 28/10/2024.

2   Koebele SV, Bimonte-Nelson HA. The endocrine-brain-aging triad where many paths meet: Female reproductive hormone changes at midlife and their influence on circuits important for learning and memory. *Experimental Gerontology.* 2017;94:14–23.
    Koebele SV, Mennenga SE, Hiroi R, et al. Cognitive changes across the menopause transition: A longitudinal evaluation of the impact of age and ovarian status on spatial memory. *Hormones and Behavior.* 2017;87:96–114.

3   Mosconi L, Berti V, Dyke J, et al. Menopause impacts human brain structure, connectivity, energy metabolism, and amyloid-beta deposition. *Scientific Reports.* 2021;11(1):10867.

4   Ibid.

5   Moseley RL, Druce T, Turner-Cobb JM. Autism research is 'all about the blokes and the kids': Autistic women breaking the silence on menopause. *British Journal of Health Psychology.* 2021;26(3):709–726.

Jenkins C, Moseley R, Matthews R, Janse Van Rensburg M, Gamble-Turner J, Brady M. 'Struggling for years': An international survey on autistic experiences of menopause. *Neurodiversity.* 2024;2:27546330241299366.

Karavidas M, de Visser RO. 'It's not just in my head, and it's not just irrelevant': Autistic negotiations of menopausal transitions. *Journal of Autism and Developmental Disorders.* 2022;52(3):1143–1155.

6   Groenman AP, Torenvliet C, Radhoe TA, Agelink van Rentergem JA, Geurts HM. Menstruation and menopause in autistic adults: Periods of importance? *Autism.* 2022;26(6):1563–1572.

7   ADDitude. ADHD impairment peaks in menopause, according to ADDitude reader survey. 2024; www.additudemag.com/menopause-symptoms-adhd-survey. Accessed 28/10/2024.

8   Johnson H, Ogden J. Much more than a biological phenomenon: A qualitative study of women's experiences of brain fog across their reproductive journey. *Journal of Health Psychology.* 2024;30(8):13591053241290656.

9   Moseley RL, Druce T, Turner-Cobb JM. Unpublished supplementary data from 'Autism research is "all about the blokes and the kids": Autistic women breaking the silence on menopause.' (2021, *British Journal of Health Psychology*).

10   O'Neill M, Jones V, Reid A. Impact of menopausal symptoms on work and careers: A cross-sectional study. *Occupational Medicine.* 2023;73(6):332–338.

Faubion SS, Enders F, Hedges MS, et al. Impact of menopause symptoms on women in the workplace. *Mayo Clinical Proceedings.* 2023;98(6):833–845.

11   Moseley RL, Druce T, Turner-Cobb JM. Autism research is 'all about the blokes and the kids': Autistic women breaking the silence on menopause. *British Journal of Health Psychology.* 2021;26(3):709–726.

Gellini H, Marczak M. 'I always knew I was different': Experiences of receiving a diagnosis of autistic spectrum disorder in adulthood – a meta-ethnographic systematic review. *Review Journal of Autism and Developmental Disorders.* 2023;11(3):620–639.

12   Moseley RL, Druce T, Turner-Cobb JM. Autism research is 'all about the blokes and the kids': Autistic women breaking the silence on menopause. *British Journal of Health Psychology.* 2021;26(3):709–726.

Brady MJ, Jenkins CA, Gamble-Turner JM, Moseley RL, Janse van Rensburg M, Matthews RJ. 'A perfect storm': Autistic experiences of menopause and midlife. *Autism.* 2024;28(6):1405–1418.

Gottardello D, Steffan B. Fundamental intersectionality of menopause and neurodivergence experiences at work. *Maturitas.* 2024;189:108107.

13   Moseley RL, Druce T, Turner-Cobb JM. Autism research is 'all about the blokes and the kids': Autistic women breaking the silence on menopause. *British Journal of Health Psychology.* 2021;26(3):709–726 (p.717).

14   Moseley RL, Druce T, Turner-Cobb JM. Unpublished supplementary data from 'Autism research is "all about the blokes and the kids": Autistic women breaking the silence on menopause.' (2021, *British Journal of Health Psychology*).

15   Brady MJ, Jenkins CA, Gamble-Turner JM, Moseley RL, Janse van Rensburg M, Matthews RJ. 'A perfect storm': Autistic experiences of menopause and midlife. *Autism.* 2024;28(6):1405–1418 (p.1411).

16   Gottardello D, Steffan B. Fundamental intersectionality of menopause and neurodivergence experiences at work. *Maturitas.* 2024;189:108107 (p.5).

17   Moseley RL, Druce T, Turner-Cobb JM. Unpublished supplementary data from 'Autism research is "all about the blokes and the kids": Autistic women breaking the silence on menopause.' (2021, *British Journal of Health Psychology*).

18   Ibid.

19   Ibid.

CHAPTER 15

1   Parenteau CI, Lampinen LL, Ghods SS, et al. Self-reported everyday sources of happiness and unhappiness in autistic adults. *Journal of Autism and Developmental Disorders.* 2023;54(4):1538–1548.

2   Whelpley CE, May CP. Seeing is disliking: Evidence of bias against individuals with autism spectrum disorder in traditional job interviews. *Journal of Autism and Developmental Disorders.* 2023;53(4):1363–1374.

Clin E, Kissine M. Neurotypical, but not autistic, adults might experience distress when looking at someone avoiding eye contact: A live face-to-face paradigm. *Autism.* 2023;27(7):1949–1959.

3   Bradley L, Shaw R, Baron-Cohen S, Cassidy S. Autistic adults' experiences of camouflaging and its perceived impact on mental health. *Autism in Adulthood.* 2021;3(4):320–329.

Evans JA, Krumrei-Mancuso EJ, Rouse SV. What you are hiding could be hurting you: Autistic masking in relation to mental health, interpersonal trauma, authenticity, and self-esteem. *Autism in Adulthood.* 2024;6(2):229–240.

4   Shalev I, Warrier V, Greenberg DM, et al. Reexamining empathy in autism: Empathic dis-equilibrium as a novel predictor of autism diagnosis and autistic traits. *Autism Research.* 2022;15(10):1917–1928.
5   Moseley R, Shalev I, Gregory N, Uzefovsky F. Empathic disequilibrium as a predictor of non-suicidal self-injury in autistic and non-autistic people. *Autism in Adulthood.* 2024.
6   Moseley RL, Druce T, Turner-Cobb J. 'When my autism broke': A qualitative study spot-lighting autistic voices on menopause. *Autism.* 2020;24(6):1423–1437.
       Moseley RL, Druce T, Turner-Cobb JM. Autism research is 'all about the blokes and the kids': Autistic women breaking the silence on menopause. *British Journal of Health Psychology.* 2021;26(3):709–726.
7   Moseley RL, Druce T, Turner-Cobb JM. Unpublished supplementary data from 'Autism research is "all about the blokes and the kids": Autistic women breaking the silence on menopause.' (2021, *British Journal of Health Psychology*).
8   Ibid.
9   Moseley RL, Druce T, Turner-Cobb JM. Autism research is 'all about the blokes and the kids': Autistic women breaking the silence on menopause. *British Journal of Health Psychology.* 2021;26(3):709–726.
10   Cook J, Crane L, Hull L, Bourne L, Mandy W. Self-reported camouflaging behaviours used by autistic adults during everyday social interactions. *Autism.* 2022;26(2):406–421.
11   Ibid.
12   Moseley RL, Druce T, Turner-Cobb JM. Autism research is 'all about the blokes and the kids': Autistic women breaking the silence on menopause. *British Journal of Health Psychology.* 2021;26(3):709–726 (p.715).

CHAPTER 16

1   Sibeoni J, Massoutier L, Valette M, et al. The sensory experiences of autistic people: A metasynthesis. *Autism.* 2022;26(5):1032–1045.
       Kirby AV, Bilder DA, Wiggins LD, et al. Sensory features in autism: Findings from a large population-based surveillance system. *Autism Research.* 2022;15(4):751–760.
2   He JL, Williams ZJ, Harris A, et al. A working taxonomy for describing the sensory differ-ences of autism. *Molecular Autism.* 2023;14(1):15.
3   Ibid.
       Lane SJ, Leão MA, Spielmann V. Sleep, sensory integration/processing, and autism: A scoping review. *Frontiers in Psychology.* 2022;13:877527.
4   MacLennan K, O'Brien S, Tavassoli T. In our own words: The complex sensory experiences of autistic adults. *Journal of Autism and Developmental Disorders.* 2021;52(7):3061–3075.
       Chen Y, Xi Z, Saunders R, Simmons D, Totsika V, Mandy W. A systematic review and meta-analysis of the relationship between sensory processing differences and internalising/externalising problems in autism. *Clinical Psychology Review.* 2024;114:102516.
5   Taels L, Feyaerts J, Lizon M, De Smet M, Vanheule S. 'I felt like my senses were under attack': An interpretative phenomenological analysis of experiences of hypersensitivity in autistic individuals. *Autism.* 2023;27(8):2269–2280 (p.2269).
6   Aloufi N, Heinrich A, Marshall K, Kluk K. Sex differences and the effect of female sex hormones on auditory function: A systematic review. *Frontiers in Human Neuroscience.* 2023;17:1077409.
7   Harper JC, Phillips S, Biswakarma R, et al. An online survey of perimenopausal women to determine their attitudes and knowledge of the menopause. *Women's Health.* 2022;18:17455057221106890.
       O'Reilly K, McDermid F, McInnes S, Peters K. An exploration of women's knowledge and experience of perimenopause and menopause: An integrative literature review. *Journal of Clinical Nursing.* 2023;32(15–16):4528–4540.
       Currie H, Moger SJ. Menopause – understanding the impact on women and their part-ners. *Post Reproductive Health.* 2019;25(4):183–190.
8   Farage MA, Osborn TW, MacLean AB. Cognitive, sensory, and emotional changes associated with the menstrual cycle: A review. *Archives of Gynecology and Obstetrics.* 2008;278:299–307.
9   Aloufi N, Heinrich A, Marshall K, Kluk K. Sex differences and the effect of female sex hormones on auditory function: A systematic review. *Frontiers in Human Neuroscience.* 2023;17:1077409.
       Al-Mana D, Ceranic B, Djahanbakhch O, Luxon L. Hormones and the auditory system: A review of physiology and pathophysiology. *Neuroscience.* 2008;153(4):881–900.
10   Albaugh SL, Wu LL, Zhang D, et al. Olfaction in pregnancy: Systematic review and meta-anal-ysis. *Chemical Senses.* 2022;47:bjac035.
       Singh AK, Agarwal M, Jain N, Garg N, Verma P, Mittal S. Effect of menopause on olfac-tory function. *National Journal of Physiology, Pharmacy and Pharmacology.* 2019;9(7):621–621.

11 Moseley RL, Druce T, Turner-Cobb JM. Autism research is 'all about the blokes and the kids': Autistic women breaking the silence on menopause. *British Journal of Health Psychology.* 2021;26(3):709–726 (p.718).

12 Moseley RL, Druce T, Turner-Cobb JM. Unpublished supplementary data from 'Autism research is "all about the blokes and the kids": Autistic women breaking the silence on menopause.' (2021, *British Journal of Health Psychology*).

13 Moseley RL, Druce T, Turner-Cobb JM. Autism research is 'all about the blokes and the kids': Autistic women breaking the silence on menopause. *British Journal of Health Psychology.* 2021;26(3):709–726 (p.718).

14 Al-Mana D, Ceranic B, Djahanbakhch O, Luxon L. Hormones and the auditory system: A review of physiology and pathophysiology. *Neuroscience.* 2008;153(4):881–900.

15 MacLennan K, O'Brien S, Tavassoli T. In our own words: The complex sensory experiences of autistic adults. *Journal of Autism and Developmental Disorders.* 2021;52(7):3061–3075.

　Harrold A, Keating K, Larkin F, Setti A. The association between sensory processing and stress in the adult population: A systematic review. *Applied Psychology: Health and Well-Being.* 2024;16(4):2536–2566.

16 Lane SJ, Leão MA, Spielmann V. Sleep, sensory integration/processing, and autism: A scoping review. *Frontiers in Psychology.* 2022;13:877527.

17 MacLennan K, Woolley C, Emily@21andsensory, et al. 'It is a big spider web of things': Sensory experiences of autistic adults in public spaces. *Autism in Adulthood.* 2022;5(4):411–422.

18 Ibid. p.411.

CHAPTER 17

1 Moseley RL, Druce T, Turner-Cobb J. 'When my autism broke': A qualitative study spotlighting autistic voices on menopause. *Autism.* 2020;24(6):1423–1437.

　Moseley RL, Druce T, Turner-Cobb JM. Autism research is 'all about the blokes and the kids': Autistic women breaking the silence on menopause. *British Journal of Health Psychology.* 2021;26(3):709–726.

　Brady MJ, Jenkins CA, Gamble-Turner JM, Moseley RL, Janse van Rensburg M, Matthews RJ. 'A perfect storm': Autistic experiences of menopause and midlife. *Autism.* 2024;28(6):1405–1418.

　Jenkins C, Moseley R, Matthews R, Janse Van Rensburg M, Gamble-Turner J, Brady M. 'Struggling for years': An international survey on autistic experiences of menopause. *Neurodiversity.* 2024;2:27546330241299366.

　Karavidas M, de Visser RO. 'It's not just in my head, and it's not just irrelevant': Autistic negotiations of menopausal transitions. *Journal of Autism and Developmental Disorders.* 2022;52(3):1143–1155.

2 Süss H, Ehlert U. Psychological resilience during the perimenopause. *Maturitas.* 2020;131:48–56.

3 Cai RY, Gibbs V, Love A, Robinson A, Fung L, Brown L. 'Self-compassion changed my life': The self-compassion experiences of autistic and non-autistic adults and its relationship with mental health and psychological wellbeing. *Journal of Autism and Developmental Disorders.* 2023;53(3):1066–1081.

4 Neville F, Sedgewick F, McClean S, White J, Bray I. Reacting, retreating, regulating, and reconnecting: How autistic adults in the United Kingdom use time alone for well-being. *Autism in Adulthood.* 2024 (p.6). https://doi.org/10.1089/aut.2024.0148

5 Long R-EM. Access points: Understanding special interests through autistic narratives. *Autism in Adulthood.* 2024. 7(1), 100–111.

6 Moseley RL, Druce T, Turner-Cobb J. 'When my autism broke': A qualitative study spotlighting autistic voices on menopause. *Autism.* 2020;24(6):1423–1437.

　Brady MJ, Jenkins CA, Gamble-Turner JM, Moseley RL, Janse van Rensburg M, Matthews RJ. 'A perfect storm': Autistic experiences of menopause and midlife. *Autism.* 2024;28(6):1405–1418.

7 Lu J, Li K, Zheng X, et al. Prevalence of menopausal symptoms and attitudes towards menopausal hormone therapy in women aged 40–60 years: A cross-sectional study. *BMC Women's Health.* 2023;23(1):472.

　Barber K, Charles A. Barriers to accessing effective treatment and support for menopausal symptoms: A qualitative study capturing the behaviours, beliefs and experiences of key stakeholders. *Patient Preference and Adherence.* 2023;17:2971–2980.

8 Panay N, Ang SB, Cheshire R, et al. Menopause and MHT in 2024: Addressing the key controversies – an International Menopause Society White Paper. *South African General Practitioner.* 2024;5(3):119–134.

9 Moseley RL, Druce T, Turner-Cobb JM. Autism research is 'all about the blokes and the kids': Autistic women breaking the silence on menopause. *British Journal of Health Psychology.* 2021;26(3):709–726.

Karavidas M, de Visser RO. 'It's not just in my head, and it's not just irrelevant': Autistic negotiations of menopausal transitions. *Journal of Autism and Developmental Disorders.* 2022;52(3):1143–1155.

Piper MA, Charlton RA. Common and unique menopause experiences among autistic and non-autistic people: A qualitative study. *Journal of Health Psychology.* 2025 (online ahead of print):13591053251316500.

10 Panay N, Ang SB, Cheshire R, et al. Menopause and MHT in 2024: Addressing the key controversies – an International Menopause Society White Paper. *South African General Practitioner.* 2024;5(3):119–134.

11 Shaw SC, Carravallah L, Johnson M, et al. Barriers to healthcare and a 'triple empathy problem' may lead to adverse outcomes for autistic adults: A qualitative study. *Autism.* 2024;28(7):13623613231205629.

12 Nicolaidis C, Raymaker D, McDonald K, et al. The development and evaluation of an online healthcare toolkit for autistic adults and their primary care providers. *Journal of General Internal Medicine.* 2016;31:1180–1189.

13 Barber K, Charles A. Barriers to accessing effective treatment and support for menopausal symptoms: A qualitative study capturing the behaviours, beliefs and experiences of key stakeholders. *Patient Preference and Adherence.* 2023;17:2971–2980.

14 Nicolaidis C, Raymaker D, McDonald K, et al. The development and evaluation of an online healthcare toolkit for autistic adults and their primary care providers. *Journal of General Internal Medicine.* 2016;31:1180–1189.

15 Moseley RL, Druce T, Turner-Cobb JM. Unpublished supplementary data from 'Autism research is "all about the blokes and the kids": Autistic women breaking the silence on menopause.' (2021, *British Journal of Health Psychology*).

16 Moseley RL, Druce T, Turner-Cobb JM. Autism research is 'all about the blokes and the kids': Autistic women breaking the silence on menopause. *British Journal of Health Psychology.* 2021;26(3):709–726.

Jenkins C, Moseley R, Matthews R, Janse Van Rensburg M, Gamble-Turner J, Brady M. 'Struggling for years': An international survey on autistic experiences of menopause. *Neurodiversity.* 2024;2:27546330241299366.

17 Moseley RL, Druce T, Turner-Cobb JM. Autism research is 'all about the blokes and the kids': Autistic women breaking the silence on menopause. *British Journal of Health Psychology.* 2021;26(3):709–726.

Brady MJ, Jenkins CA, Gamble-Turner JM, Moseley RL, Janse van Rensburg M, Matthews RJ. 'A perfect storm': Autistic experiences of menopause and midlife. *Autism.* 2024;28(6):1405–1418.

Jenkins C, Moseley R, Matthews R, Janse Van Rensburg M, Gamble-Turner J, Brady M. 'Struggling for years': An international survey on autistic experiences of menopause. *Neurodiversity.* 2024;2:27546330241299366.

18 Watts G, Crompton C, Grainger C, et al. 'A certain magic' – autistic adults' experiences of interacting with other autistic people and its relation to Quality of Life: A systematic review and thematic meta-synthesis. *Autism.* 2024;29(9):13623613241255811 (p.6).

19 Moseley RL, Druce T, Turner-Cobb JM. Unpublished supplementary data from 'Autism research is "all about the blokes and the kids": Autistic women breaking the silence on menopause.' (2021, *British Journal of Health Psychology*).

20 Moseley RL, Druce T, Turner-Cobb JM. Autism research is 'all about the blokes and the kids': Autistic women breaking the silence on menopause. *British Journal of Health Psychology.* 2021;26(3):709–726 (p.760).

CHAPTER 18

1 Moseley RL, Druce T, Turner-Cobb JM. Autism research is 'all about the blokes and the kids': Autistic women breaking the silence on menopause. *British Journal of Health Psychology.* 2021;26(3):709–726.

2 Harper JC, Phillips S, Biswakarma R, et al. An online survey of perimenopausal women to determine their attitudes and knowledge of the menopause. *Women's Health.* 2022;18:17455057221106890.

Tariq B, Phillips S, Biswakarma R, Talaulikar V, Harper JC. Women's knowledge and attitudes to the menopause: A comparison of women over 40 who were in the perimenopause, post menopause and those not in the peri or post menopause. *BMC Women's Health.* 2023;23(1):460.

Ray E, Maybin JA, Harper JC. Perimenopausal women's voices: How does their period at the end of reproductive life affect wellbeing? *Post Reproductive Health.* 2023;29(4):201–221.

Hickey M, LaCroix AZ, Doust J, et al. An empowerment model for managing menopause. *The Lancet.* 2024;403(10430):947–957.

3   Moseley RL, Druce T, Turner-Cobb JM. Autism research is 'all about the blokes and the kids': Autistic women breaking the silence on menopause. *British Journal of Health Psychology.* 2021;26(3):709–726.
    Jenkins C, Moseley R, Matthews R, Janse Van Rensburg M, Gamble-Turner J, Brady M. 'Struggling for years': An international survey on autistic experiences of menopause. *Neurodiversity.* 2024;2:27546330241299366.

4   Moseley RL, Druce T, Turner-Cobb JM. Unpublished supplementary data from 'Autism research is "all about the blokes and the kids": Autistic women breaking the silence on menopause.' (2021, *British Journal of Health Psychology*).

5   Galambos NL, Krahn HJ, Johnson MD, Lachman ME. The U shape of happiness across the life course: Expanding the discussion. *Perspectives on Psychological Science.* 2020;15(4):898–912.

6   Aitken R, Berry K, Gowen E, Brown L. How do autistic adults experience ageing? A qualitative interview study. Unpublished manuscript, Open Science Framework, 2024.
    Ommensen B, Sofronoff K, Attwood T, Pachana N. 'Life's good now': The paradox of poignancy and positivity in autistic ageing. 2005: https://doi.org/10.31234/osf.io/856xc_v2

7   Ommensen B, Sofronoff K, Attwood T, Pachana N. 'Life's good now': The paradox of poignancy and positivity in autistic ageing. 2005: https://doi.org/10.31234/osf.io/856xc_v2.

8   Moseley RL, Druce T, Turner-Cobb JM. Autism research is 'all about the blokes and the kids': Autistic women breaking the silence on menopause. *British Journal of Health Psychology.* 2021;26(3):709–726 (p.716).

9   Jenkins C, Moseley R, Matthews R, Janse Van Rensburg M, Gamble-Turner J, Brady M. 'Struggling for years': An international survey on autistic experiences of menopause. *Neurodiversity.* 2024;2:27546330241299366 (p.11).

10 Jakubowski KP, Barinas-Mitchell E, Chang Y-F, Maki PM, Matthews KA, Thurston RC. The cardiovascular cost of silence: Relationships between self-silencing and carotid atherosclerosis in midlife women. *Annals of Behavioral Medicine.* 2022;56(3):282–290.

11 Moseley RL, Druce T, Turner-Cobb JM. Autism research is 'all about the blokes and the kids': Autistic women breaking the silence on menopause. *British Journal of Health Psychology.* 2021;26(3):709–726.
    Jenkins C, Moseley R, Matthews R, Janse Van Rensburg M, Gamble-Turner J, Brady M. 'Struggling for years': An international survey on autistic experiences of menopause. *Neurodiversity.* 2024;2:27546330241299366.

12 Jenkins C, Moseley R, Matthews R, Janse Van Rensburg M, Gamble-Turner J, Brady M. 'Struggling for years': An international survey on autistic experiences of menopause. *Neurodiversity.* 2024;2:27546330241299366 (p.11).

13 Moseley RL, Druce T, Turner-Cobb JM. Unpublished supplementary data from 'Autism research is "all about the blokes and the kids": Autistic women breaking the silence on menopause.' (2021, *British Journal of Health Psychology*).

14 Moseley RL, Druce T, Turner-Cobb JM. Autism research is 'all about the blokes and the kids': Autistic women breaking the silence on menopause. *British Journal of Health Psychology.* 2021;26(3):709–726.
    Karavidas M, de Visser RO. 'It's not just in my head, and it's not just irrelevant': Autistic negotiations of menopausal transitions. *Journal of Autism and Developmental Disorders.* 2022;52(3):1143–1155.
    Piper MA, Charlton RA. Common and unique menopause experiences among autistic and non-autistic people: A qualitative study. *Journal of Health Psychology.* 2025 (online ahead of print):13591053251316500.

15 Steward R, Crane L, Mairi Roy E, Remington A, Pellicano E. 'Life is much more difficult to manage during periods': Autistic experiences of menstruation. *Journal of Autism and Developmental Disorders.* 2018;48(12):4287–4292.
    Gray LJ, Durand H. Experiences of dysmenorrhea and its treatment among allistic and autistic menstruators: A thematic analysis. *BMC Women's Health.* 2023;23(1):1–13.

16 Moseley RL, Druce T, Turner-Cobb JM. Unpublished supplementary data from 'Autism research is "all about the blokes and the kids": Autistic women breaking the silence on menopause.' (2021, *British Journal of Health Psychology*).

17 Ibid.

18 Ibid.

19 Moseley RL, Druce T, Turner-Cobb JM. Unpublished supplementary data from 'Autism research is "all about the blokes and the kids": Autistic women breaking the silence on menopause.' (2021, *British Journal of Health Psychology*).
    Jenkins C, Moseley R, Matthews R, Janse Van Rensburg M, Gamble-Turner J, Brady M. 'Struggling for years': An international survey on autistic experiences of menopause. *Neurodiversity.* 2024;2:27546330241299366.

20 Moseley RL, Druce T, Turner-Cobb JM. Autism research is 'all about the blokes and the kids': Autistic women breaking the silence on menopause. *British Journal of Health Psychology.* 2021;26(3):709–726.

21 Moseley RL, Druce T, Turner-Cobb JM. Unpublished supplementary data from 'Autism research is "all about the blokes and the kids": Autistic women breaking the silence on menopause.' (2021, *British Journal of Health Psychology*).

CHAPTER 19

1 Harlow SD, Gass M, Hall JE, et al. Executive summary of the Stages of Reproductive Aging Workshop + 10: Addressing the unfinished agenda of staging reproductive aging. *Climacteric.* 2012;15(2):105–114.

2 Davis SR, Lambrinoudaki I, Lumsden M, et al. Menopause (Primer). *Nature Reviews: Disease Primers.* 2015;1:15004.

3 Politi MC, Schleinitz MD, Col NF. Revisiting the duration of vasomotor symptoms of menopause: A meta-analysis. *Journal of General Internal Medicine.* 2008;23:1507–1513.
     Blümel J, Chedraui P, Baron G, et al. Menopausal symptoms appear before the menopause and persist 5 years beyond: A detailed analysis of a multinational study. *Climacteric.* 2012;15(6):542–551.

4 Hachul H, Bittencourt LRA, Soares Jr JM, Tufik S, Baracat EC. Sleep in post-menopausal women: Differences between early and late post-menopause. *European Journal of Obstetrics & Gynecology and Reproductive Biology.* 2009;145(1):81–84.

5 Harlow SD, Gass M, Hall JE, et al. Executive summary of the Stages of Reproductive Aging Workshop + 10: Addressing the unfinished agenda of staging reproductive aging. *Climacteric.* 2012;15(2):105–114.

6 Aitken R, Berry K, Gowen E, Brown L. How do autistic adults experience ageing? A qualitative interview study. Unpublished manuscript, Open Science Framework, 2024 (p.12).

7 Moseley RL, Druce T, Turner-Cobb JM. Autism research is 'all about the blokes and the kids': Autistic women breaking the silence on menopause. *British Journal of Health Psychology.* 2021;26(3):709–726.
     Jenkins C, Moseley R, Matthews R, Janse Van Rensburg M, Gamble-Turner J, Brady M. 'Struggling for years': An international survey on autistic experiences of menopause. *Neurodiversity.* 2024;2:27546330241299366.

8 Moseley RL, Druce T, Turner-Cobb JM. Unpublished supplementary data from 'Autism research is "all about the blokes and the kids": Autistic women breaking the silence on menopause.' (2021, *British Journal of Health Psychology*).

9 Moseley RL, Druce T, Turner-Cobb JM. Autism research is 'all about the blokes and the kids': Autistic women breaking the silence on menopause. *British Journal of Health Psychology.* 2021;26(3):709–726 (p.719).

CHAPTER 20

1 Moseley RL, Druce T, Turner-Cobb JM. Autism research is 'all about the blokes and the kids': Autistic women breaking the silence on menopause. *British Journal of Health Psychology.* 2021;26(3):709–726.
     Brady MJ, Jenkins CA, Gamble-Turner JM, Moseley RL, Janse van Rensburg M, Matthews RJ. 'A perfect storm': Autistic experiences of menopause and midlife. *Autism.* 2024;28(6):1405–1418.
     Jenkins C, Moseley R, Matthews R, Janse Van Rensburg M, Gamble-Turner J, Brady M. 'Struggling for years': An international survey on autistic experiences of menopause. *Neurodiversity.* 2024;2:27546330241299366.
     Karavidas M, de Visser RO. 'It's not just in my head, and it's not just irrelevant': Autistic negotiations of menopausal transitions. *Journal of Autism and Developmental Disorders.* 2022;52(3):1143–1155.
     Piper MA, Charlton RA. Common and unique menopause experiences among autistic and non-autistic people: A qualitative study. *Journal of Health Psychology.* 2025 (online ahead of print):13591053251316500.
     Nicolaidis C, Raymaker D, McDonald K, et al. The development and evaluation of an online healthcare toolkit for autistic adults and their primary care providers. *Journal of General Internal Medicine.* 2016;31:1180–1189.

2 Martin-Key NA, Funnell EL, Spadaro B, Bahn S. Perceptions of healthcare provision throughout the menopause in the UK: A mixed-methods study. *npj Women's Health.* 2023;1(1):2.
     Panay N, Ang SB, Cheshire R, et al. Menopause and MHT in 2024: Addressing the key controversies – an International Menopause Society White Paper. *South African General Practitioner.* 2024;5(3):119–134.

3   Nicolaidis C, Raymaker D, McDonald K, et al. The development and evaluation of an online healthcare toolkit for autistic adults and their primary care providers. *Journal of General Internal Medicine.* 2016;31:1180–1189.

4   Corden K, Brewer R, Cage E. A systematic review of healthcare professionals' knowledge, self-efficacy and attitudes towards working with autistic people. *Review Journal of Autism and Developmental Disorders.* 2022;9(3):386–399.

     Urbanowicz A, Parkin T, van Dooren K, Girdler S, Ciccarelli M, Lennox N. The experiences, views, and needs of health professionals who provide care to adults on the autism spectrum. *Research and Practice in Intellectual and Developmental Disabilities.* 2020;7(2):179–192.

5   Moseley RL, Druce T, Turner-Cobb JM. Autism research is 'all about the blokes and the kids': Autistic women breaking the silence on menopause. *British Journal of Health Psychology.* 2021;26(3):709–726.

     Brady MJ, Jenkins CA, Gamble-Turner JM, Moseley RL, Janse van Rensburg M, Matthews RJ. 'A perfect storm': Autistic experiences of menopause and midlife. *Autism.* 2024;28(6):1405–1418.

     Karavidas M, de Visser RO. 'It's not just in my head, and it's not just irrelevant': Autistic negotiations of menopausal transitions. *Journal of Autism and Developmental Disorders.* 2022;52(3):1143–1155.

     Piper MA, Charlton RA. Common and unique menopause experiences among autistic and non-autistic people: A qualitative study. *Journal of Health Psychology.* 2025 (online ahead of print):13591053251316500.

     Grove R, Clapham H, Moodie T, Gurrin S, Hall G. 'Living in a world that's not about us': The impact of everyday life on the health and wellbeing of autistic women and gender diverse people. *Women's Health.* 2023;19:17455057231189542.

     de Visser RO, Moseley R, Gamble-Turner J, et al. Unmet need for autism-aware care for gynaecological, menstrual and sexual wellbeing. *Autism.* 2024;29(4):934–944.

     Miller KHK, Cooper DS, Song W, Shea LL. Self-reported service needs and barriers reported by autistic adults: Differences by gender identity. *Research in Autism Spectrum Disorders.* 2022;92:101916.

6   Mansour H, Gillions A, Brown J, et al. 'It's designed for someone who is not me': A reflexive thematic analysis of the unmet healthcare support needs in UK autistic adults aged 65 years and over. *Autism.* 2024;29(3):13623613241291081.

7   Moseley RL, Druce T, Turner-Cobb JM. Autism research is 'all about the blokes and the kids': Autistic women breaking the silence on menopause. *British Journal of Health Psychology.* 2021;26(3):709–726.

     Brady MJ, Jenkins CA, Gamble-Turner JM, Moseley RL, Janse van Rensburg M, Matthews RJ. 'A perfect storm': Autistic experiences of menopause and midlife. *Autism.* 2024;28(6):1405–1418.

     Radev S, Freeth M, Thompson ARJA. How healthcare systems are experienced by autistic adults in the United Kingdom: A meta-ethnography. *Autism.* 2024;28(9): 2166–2178.

     Moseley R, Marsden S, Allison C, et al. Suicidality in autistic people: A mixed-methods approach to contributing factors. Unpublished manuscript, ResearchGate, 2025.

8   Nicolaidis C, Raymaker D, McDonald K, et al. The development and evaluation of an online healthcare toolkit for autistic adults and their primary care providers. *Journal of General Internal Medicine.* 2016;31:1180–1189.

9   Moseley RL, Druce T, Turner-Cobb JM. Autism research is 'all about the blokes and the kids': Autistic women breaking the silence on menopause. *British Journal of Health Psychology.* 2021;26(3):709–726.

     Brady MJ, Jenkins CA, Gamble-Turner JM, Moseley RL, Janse van Rensburg M, Matthews RJ. 'A perfect storm': Autistic experiences of menopause and midlife. *Autism.* 2024;28(6):1405–1418.

     Jenkins C, Moseley R, Matthews R, Janse Van Rensburg M, Gamble-Turner J, Brady M. 'Struggling for years': An international survey on autistic experiences of menopause. *Neurodiversity.* 2024;2:27546330241299366.

10   Nicolaidis C, Raymaker D, McDonald K, et al. The development and evaluation of an online healthcare toolkit for autistic adults and their primary care providers. *Journal of General Internal Medicine.* 2016;31:1180–1189.

11   Ye M, Shou M, Zhang J, et al. Efficacy of cognitive therapy and behavior therapy for menopausal symptoms: A systematic review and meta-analysis. *Psychological Medicine.* 2022;52(3):433–445.

12   Brede J, Cage E, Trott J, et al. 'We have to try to find a way, a clinical bridge' – autistic adults' experience of accessing and receiving support for mental health difficulties: A systematic review and thematic meta-synthesis. *Clinical Psychology Review.* 2022;93:102131.

13   Bulluss E. Therapist cultural humility is a crucial component of psychotherapy with autistic clients. *The Science of Psychotherapy.* 2021;5(6):46–50.

14   Benevides TW, Cook B, Klinger LG, et al. Brief report: Under-identification of symptomatic menopause in publicly-insured autistic people. *Journal of Autism and Developmental Disorders.* 2024: doi 10.1007/s10803-024-06516-x.
15   Brady MJ, Jenkins CA, Gamble-Turner JM, Moseley RL, Janse van Rensburg M, Matthews RJ. 'A perfect storm': Autistic experiences of menopause and midlife. *Autism.* 2024;28(6):1405–1418 (p.1412).
16   Malone KM, Pearson JN, Palazzo KN, Manns LD, Rivera AQ, Mason Martin DL. The scholarly neglect of Black autistic adults in autism research. *Autism in Adulthood.* 2022 (p.273).

CHAPTER 21

1   O'Nions E, Lewer D, Petersen I, et al. Estimating life expectancy and years of life lost for autistic people in the UK: A matched cohort study. *Lancet Regional Health – Europe.* 2024;36:100776.
      Ward JH, Weir E, Allison C, Baron-Cohen S. Increased rates of chronic physical health conditions across all organ systems in autistic adolescents and adults. *Molecular Autism.* 2023;14(1):35.
      Weir E, Allison C, Warrier V, Baron-Cohen S. Increased prevalence of non-communicable physical health conditions among autistic adults. *Autism.* 2021;25(3):681–694.
      Santomauro DF, Hedley D, Sahin E, et al. The global burden of suicide mortality among people on the autism spectrum: A systematic review, meta-analysis, and extension of estimates from the Global Burden of Disease Study 2021. *Psychiatry Research.* 2024;341:116150.
2   National Autistic Society. Joint call to end an 'avoidable and devastating crisis' of autism diagnosis waiting times. 2024, 25 October. www.autism.org.uk/what-we-do/news/joint-call. Accessed 14/01/2025.

Index

ADHD
  and autism 102–3, 105–7
  and menopause 101–7
  and people of colour 110
  and queer people 112
alexithymia 68, 83, 102, 132, 154–5
alternative treatments 181–2
anger issues 133–5
anxiety 133–5
attention spans 139–42
attitudes towards menopause
  44–6
autism
  and ADHD 102–3, 105–7
  diagnosis of 22, 89–97
  and learning disabilities 99–101
  as positive identity 14–15
  understanding neurodivergent
    status 22
autism and menopause
  experiences of 62–4
  impact of physical changes 125–7
  information access 75–6
  and people of colour 110–12
  poorer mental health 74–5
  poorer physical health 74
  and queer people 112–16
  struggles with change 67–8
  struggles with cognitive
    processes 68–9

struggles with emotions 68
struggles with low self-
  worth 72–3
struggles with periods 73–4
struggles with physical
  symptoms 70–1
support for 76–7
traumatic pasts 77–8
awareness of menopause 21–2

biology of menopause 24–5
body shape changes 123–4
brain fog 38, 142–5

children 81–3
cognitive dysfunction
  38, 142–5, 147–8
cognitive processes
  and attention spans 139–42
  autism and menopause 68–9
  and brain fog 38, 142–5
    and cognitive dysfunction
    38, 142–5, 147–8
  everyday impacts of
    dysfunction 147–8
  help with 148–9
  and memory 139–42
  and work-related
    challenges 145–6
Common-Sense Model 45

communication issues
  masking 152–60
  quotes on 150–2
  social communication 152–60

diagnosis of autism 22
  before menopause 94–7
  of girls and women 90–1
  masking of autism 93
  undiagnosed lives 91–2
Diagnostic and Statistical
    Manual of Mental
    Disorders (DSM) 89, 90
duration of menopause 20–1

early menopause 29
education on menopause 21–2
emotional reactivity 130–2
emotions
  and alexithymia 68, 83,
      102, 132, 154–5
  anger issues 133–5
  and anxiety 133–5
  autism and menopause 68
  and depression 133–5
  and emotional reactivity 130–2
  positive changes 135–7
  quotes on 129–30
      symptoms of menopause 38

Fawcett Society 39

headaches 38–9
health
  during and after
      menopause 56–9
  in midlife 87–8
  poorer physical health 74
  stress impacts on 52–6
healthcare providers
  advice for 201–12

and management of
    menopause 180–1
hormonal changes 30–3, 165
hormone replacement
    therapy (HRT) 179–80
hot flushes 36–8, 70–1, 121
hypersensitivity 164–5
hyposensitivity 163–4

information on menopause
  autistic people 75–6
  management of menopause 178
  psychology of menopause 42–4
      understanding
      menopause 21–2
intersectionality 108–10

joint stiffness/pain 124–5

knowledge of menopause 42–4

Lachman, M. 47, 48, 82
Langer-Shapland, K. 100
language of menopause 14, 27–8
learning disabilities 99–101
low self-worth 72–3

management of menopause
  alternative treatments for 181–2
  coping skills for 176–7
  healthcare providers 180–1
  hormone replacement
      therapy (HRT) 179–80
  information on menopause 178
  and menopausal transition 173–4
  preparations for 172–3
  self-care 174–6
  social support for 182–3
masking 93, 152–60
memory 139–42
menopausal transition

and management of
    menopause 173–4
in reproductive lifespan 27
menopause
    and ADHD 101–7
    attitudes towards 44–6
    biology of 24–5
    different experiences of 13
    hormonal changes in 30–3
    language of 14, 27–8
    and learning disabilities 99–101
    management of 171–84
    positives of 185–93
    reasons for 25–6
    in reproductive lifespan 26–9
        understanding 19–23
midlife issues
    challenges around children 81–3
    challenges of menopause 47–50
    health conditions 87–8
    parenting own parents 83–4
    relationship changes 86–7
    work-related challenges 84–6
migraines 38–9
mood swings 39

neurological symptoms 33–4
    cognitive dysfunction 38
    emotional symptoms 38
    headaches 38–9
    hot flushes 36–8
    migraines 38–9
    mood swings 39
    sleep disruption 38
    vasomotor symptoms 36–8
night sweats 121

onset of menopause 20–1, 29

parenting own parents 83–4
people of colour 110–12

perimenopause
    description of 14
    in reproductive lifespan 27
periods 73–4, 121–3, 190–1
physical symptoms of
    menopause 40, 70–1, 118–27
positive emotional changes 135–7
positives of menopause
    periods 190–1
    and relationships 189–90
    self-discovery 192–3
    slowing down 187–9
    social judgements 186–7
premenopause 27
postmenopause
    disappointments with 199–200
    experiences of 194–200
    positives of 197–8
    in reproductive lifespan 27
premature menopause 29
preparation for menopause 21–2
psychology of menopause
    impact of 41–2
    information on menopause 42–4
    knowledge of menopause 42–4
    midlife challenges 47–50
    resilience factors 46–7
    understanding of
        menopause 42–4

reasons for menopause 25–6
relationship changes 86–7, 189–90
reproductive lifespan 26–9
resilience factors 46–7

self-care 174–6
self-discovery 192–3
sensory changes
    complexities of 167–9
    experiences of 165–6
    hormonal changes 165

sensory changes *cont.*
  hypersensitivity 164–5
  hyposensitivity 163–4
  quotes on 161–3
  sensory-seeking 164
sensory-seeking 164
sleep disruption 38
slowing down 187–9
social judgements 186–7
STRAW+10 26–9
stress
  and autistic people 77–8
  impacts on health 52–4
  social support for 54–6
support
  for management of
    menopause 182–3
  for people with autism 76–8
    for stress 54–6
SWAN study 54
symptoms of menopause
  complexity of 39–40
  neurological symptoms
    33–4, 36–9
  physical symptoms 40

range of 21
severity of 21
varieties of 34–5

traumatic pasts 77–8

understanding menopause
  awareness of menopause 21–2
  duration of menopause 20–1
  education on menopause 21–2
  information on menopause 21–2
  onset of menopause 20–1, 29
  preparation for menopause 21–2
  psychology of menopause 42–4
  quotes on 19–20
  symptoms of menopause 21
undiagnosed lives 91–2

vasomotor symptoms 36–8

weight change 123–4
work-related challenges
  and cognitive dysfunction
    145–6
  in midlife 84–6